Dancing in the Rain

Dancing in the Rain

My journey of hope, courage and resilience

Amy Dowden

PIATKUS

PIATKUS

First published in Great Britain in 2024 by Piatkus

1 3 5 7 9 10 8 6 4 2

A CIP catalogue record for this book
is available from the British Library.

ISBN 978-0-349-44204-4

All photographs from the author's collection.

Typeset in Garamond by M Rules
Printed and bound in Great Britain by
Clays Ltd, Elcograf S.p.A.

Papers used by Piatkus are from well-managed forests
and other responsible sources.

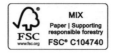

Piatkus
An imprint of
Little, Brown Book Group
Carmelite House
50 Victoria Embankment
London EC4Y 0DZ
An Hachette UK Company
www.hachette.co.uk

www.littlebrown.co.uk

For my partner in life and on the dance floor,
Ben Jones, my wonderful family, Richard, Gillian,
Lloyd and Rebecca, and all the health professionals
that have supported me over the years.

Contents

Preface

I'm in my element when I'm on the dance floor. Once the music is on and it's in my body, I just go for it – I don't care what anyone thinks. It's like that scene in the musical *Singin' in the Rain*, where Gene Kelly's character is strolling along the street during a downpour. He's got his problems, but he's feeling happy and in love; he starts humming, breaks into song and soon he's getting completely carried away, spinning his umbrella, tap-dancing on the kerb and stamping in puddles. He's not waiting for the storm to blow over, he's not bothered about getting wet. The music is in him, he's got to dance – and when he's dancing, nothing else matters. Well, that's me, too.

Dancing has got me through the roughest of times. I've had a chronic illness since the age of eleven that has led to excruciating pain, vomiting, emergency trips to hospital and a long list of other setbacks and disappointments in life. And then, in 2023, I was diagnosed with breast cancer. Knowing I've got my dancing has kept me going. It's been my saviour.

Dancing is my happy place and even just thinking about it lifts me up. When I'm laid up in bed, feeling bored and depressed, I only have to imagine a new dance move, or teaching, or being on *Strictly*, and suddenly there's a smile on my face.

But of course there are times when the tears come. When life seems unfair and I feel miserable and sorry for myself, and a whole load of other negative stuff that I don't want to be feeling. *I didn't ask for this*, I think. Isn't it bad enough that illness kept getting in the way of my dancing dreams when I was growing up? Did I have to go and get cancer now, too, stopping me doing the job I love with my best friends in the world? Did I have to find a lump in my chest the day before I went away on honeymoon? And then cope with the news when I was back that they'd found other tumours as well, that it could be difficult to have children in the future? It's more than a few raindrops – sometimes it feels like it's raining bricks on me.

How do you keep on going and trying when things are that tough? It's natural to feel down when you're faced with difficulty or uncertainty, whether it's sickness, loss, a career setback or just feeling intimidated by the future – but how do you get back up?

Well, I haven't got all the answers, I'm not going to lie. But I've had to pick myself up from the floor more than most, so I can tell you what works for me. I can tell you about the obstacles I've had to face on my journey so far, and how I've managed to overcome them and still achieve my dreams. How I've found the strength and determination to keep going and build up my resilience.

Although I'll be describing the down times along with the ups, I'm hoping this book will be inspirational for anybody who is facing challenges, large or small. And if that's you, I hope it will help you find the courage to rise up and meet them.

'Don't get bitter, get better.' That's my mantra. And it applies to everything, really.

Introduction

I only ever wanted to be known for being Amy the dancer. But life doesn't always turn out how you expect it to, does it? Out of the blue, you find yourself facing obstacles you never thought you'd come up against. You have to rethink, adjust and adapt to a completely new situation. Maybe that's why people say you learn more from the downs than the ups in life.

By the time I was thirty-two, I already had a lot of practice in dealing with the unexpected. But in April 2023 I was about to learn that lesson all over again.

It's a time that is still so vivid in my mind – the days before everything changed. I remember fizzing with happiness as I waved a thick folder of documents and printouts at Ben. 'Passports, tickets, hotel reservations . . . we're all set!'

He eyed me with amusement. I was sitting in a sea of discarded clothes on our bedroom floor, next to a suitcase spilling over with bikinis and sundresses. 'Are you sure about that?' he said.

Ben knows I love everything about going on holiday. The excitement of the days leading up to it. Going to sleep the night before and thinking, 'Tomorrow we'll be there!' Even the packing doesn't bother me – I'm just looking forward to stepping off that plane and feeling the sun on my face.

And this was our honeymoon I was packing for. It was going to be a luxury, once-in-a-lifetime holiday in the Maldives, with gorgeous food, gorgeous weather and – best of all – pure me and Ben time. That last bit was what I was looking forward to the most, because although it was nearly a year since we'd walked down the aisle together, our schedules were so busy that we hadn't had a chance to go away, just the two of us. Now, finally, the time had come. I was so excited.

But first we had to get through a busy weekend in Blackpool, where some of the formation teams from our dance academy were competing at the British Open Formation Championships. Ben and I had been teaching Latin and ballroom dancing classes for years before we real-ised our dream of starting the Art in Motion Dance Academy in 2016. Going to Blackpool with our students is one of the highlights of our year. And it was Ben's birthday while we were there, so we organised a karaoke night with the kids on the Friday, which was brilliant – especially when I got up and sang 'The Greatest Love of All' and everyone covered their ears with their hands . . .

We had an early start on the Saturday morning. The first rounds of the competition kicked off at nine o'clock and we had all the kids' hair and make-up to do beforehand. I got up and jumped in the shower, giggling at the memory of my terrible singing the night before. As the hot water pounded against my skin and woke me up, I did a check of my breasts, but only a quick one because we had a really busy day ahead. Skimming my hand over my right breast, I felt a slight swelling. Was it a lump? I didn't have time to examine it properly and hurried to get dressed, but it stayed in the back of my mind.

After two long and busy days in the ballroom, it was time to go home. At last we could unwind and get excited about going on honeymoon. 'Not long now,' Ben said, as we sped down the motorway. 'Sun, sea and cocktails . . . ' He grinned at me.

I sank into my seat with a smile. 'Hmm, can't wait.'

That night, hoping the swelling had gone, I checked my breasts properly and had a really good feel. In my right breast, I could make out a solid, oval shape that moved when I pressed it. *There is a lump*, I thought, and my heart sank.

The next day we were taking the night flight to Dubai before flying on to the Maldives. We spent the morning packing our last bits and pieces, and sorting out the house. Ben's mum was coming round and, before she arrived, I had another good feel of my breast. The lump was still there.

I didn't say anything to Ben, because I knew he would insist on going straight to the doctor, and then we'd miss our flight. And we really needed this break together. I tried to focus on the positive: I'd been secretly Googling whenever Ben wasn't looking and I'd read that around 80 per cent of breast lumps are noncancerous – they usually turn out to be a cyst or a rubbery lump called a fibroadenoma.

It's probably benign, I told myself, although deep down I knew it wasn't. My mum had been diagnosed with breast cancer when she was fifty. It was in our family.

That evening Ben and I flew off to our breathtaking resort in the Maldives, with its huge skies, turquoise seas and powdery white beaches. It was everything we'd dreamed of. It was paradise. We felt so lucky to be there.

But for me there was a shadow hanging over everything. I tried to enjoy myself, but my happiness felt like a mask. Every time I put suntan lotion on, I could feel the lump in my breast. And maybe I was imagining it, but it felt like it was getting bigger.

I still didn't say anything to Ben, but I had a really bad feeling in my gut about what it could be. All these negative thoughts were going through my mind as I lay on my sun lounger, listening to the sea gently lapping against the shore.

How long have I got? Will I be here next year?

As humans, we always fear the worst. We can never go for the positive, especially when it's a health worry. It didn't help that the position of my lump kept coming up on Google as the worst place to have it. I was reading too much and it was sending me into a panic.

'Stop worrying and make the most of this holiday,' I told myself. 'It might be the last holiday you ever have.'

I felt very alone. I really needed someone to talk to, but I couldn't bring myself to ruin Ben's holiday; I didn't want him worrying as well. Anyway, until we knew what the lump was, what good would it do? I just had to keep my fingers crossed and hope for the best.

But about halfway through our trip, I messaged a friend I'd worked with the year before: 'Hey, how you doing? How's treatment going?'

She quickly got back to me with news of her recovery. Then I asked a few questions about how she'd found her lump and what it had looked like, hoping she wouldn't realise why I was suddenly so interested. I don't think I fooled her, though, because she told me afterwards that she'd wondered if something was up.

✦

As our holiday came to an end, I started trying to figure out how I'd get to the doctor's when we got home. My schedule was absolutely crazy: we were getting back on the Wednesday in time to do a dance show on the Friday; then it was my brother Lloyd's wedding on the Saturday, which we'd been looking forward to for ages. It was also the weekend of the King's coronation and on the Monday I had the honour of presenting a live segment for the BBC. And, as it was a bank holiday weekend, I knew I wouldn't be able to get hold of my GP until the Tuesday – but on the Tuesday I would be back in Blackpool judging the World Dance Championships. That meant I wouldn't be able to see a doctor for at least a week after we got home, and the waiting was already unbearable.

My brother's wedding was gorgeous, but the lump was constantly on my mind, just screaming at me, and over the course of the day I developed a nasty cough. We saw family on the Sunday and on the Monday night I went to the Wales Millennium Centre in Cardiff to do a TV interview with one of the King's royal harpists, as part of the coronation celebrations. When she told me that she had just come out the other side of breast cancer, it felt like a sign.

On the Tuesday morning, I crept into our bedroom en suite and rang my GP's surgery. My GP rang straight back and said, 'I'll see you tomorrow.' So on the Wednesday, I drove from Blackpool to Wales, where I was scheduled to be filming in the afternoon anyway.

'I can feel a lump here,' I told the GP, when I went for my appointment, 'and I can feel a slight lump here as well.'

She was pretty chilled about it. 'Don't worry, we get loads of cysts in people your age.'

'Yes, but my mum had breast cancer,' I said.

'But she was in her fifties and you're thirty-two, so I can't see a link there. If she had been younger, I'd be worried, but I'm sure this will turn out to be nothing . . .'

She felt around for the lump and when she found it, her expression changed. She took a tape measure and noted its exact size. Then she picked up her phone and made a call. 'I need to make an emergency referral,' she said.

That call marked the beginning of one of the toughest periods of my life. But as I left the GP's surgery, I reminded myself that I'd faced tough times before. Since the age of eleven I'd had Crohn's disease, a chronic and debilitating illness that had held me back and made it even harder than it already was to make it to the top of a tough profession. I'd spent more than half my life going from one health crisis to the next, suffering indescribable pain, sickness and exhaustion, and I'd learned to live with doubt and uncertainty along the way. And because I'd experienced all of this, I knew that, with the love and support of my family and friends, I could cope with almost anything life threw at me.

So now it was time to draw on all the lessons I'd learned over the years, and on the determination and self-belief that my parents had instilled in me.

I know how to get through this, I told myself. I can do it.

Only, I felt so scared.

Chapter 1

Follow your dreams

When I was growing up, I was always being told that I wouldn't make it as a professional dancer: 'Don't be so silly. You'll never make the break into dancing.' I was just another kid, like so many others, growing up with big, out of reach dreams. I guess they were thinking: what made me so special that I could make my dreams happen?

But when someone says, 'You can't', I'll do everything to try to show them that I can. And it's especially true when it comes to dancing, because I made it my mission from a very young age that this was what I wanted to do.

I was a ball of energy when I was a child. You couldn't keep me still. My parents, Richard and Gillian Dowden, were constantly looking for ways to wear me out. My nan knew how to keep me busy, though; I didn't want to watch telly, so she'd dress me up and get me doing shows and performances in the living room with my brother, Lloyd, and twin sister, Rebecca.

'Amy's going to be on the stage,' she told my mum when I was six.

Mum smiled. 'Just as long as it keeps her occupied . . .'

◆

I discovered my love of dancing on my eighth birthday, while we were on holiday in Cornwall and staying in my granddad's static caravan. After a day spent running races and digging in the sand, my parents took me, my brother and sister up to the caravan park clubhouse to see if there was anything going on. Just to stop me bouncing off the walls, I think.

Luckily for them, the entertainment that night included a kids' disco-dancing competition, with a whole load of pop music and flashing lights to keep me distracted.

'It's time to show off your moves in the disco dance-off!' yelled the DJ.

I jumped up and rushed onto the dance floor, dragging my sister with me. 'Come on, we're doing this!'

I think Rebecca would have been happy to sit down with her popcorn and watch the contest, but she went along with it and enjoyed it in her usual easy-going way. Meanwhile, I absolutely loved it: the dancing, the spotlight, the attention, the music, the audience – everything. I bounced around throwing shapes and having the time of my life, and at the end I won a medallion that I proudly showed off to anyone and everyone for the rest of the holiday.

That was all it took to light the fuse. 'Can I go to dancing lessons? Please? Please?' I begged my parents.

Back home in Caerphilly in Wales, Rebecca and I already went to a twins club, Rainbows, swimming and other groups (see what I mean about trying to wear me out?). 'But maybe we can squeeze in one more activity,' Mum said.

They found a local dance class and signed me up, thinking it would be a great way of keeping me busy for £2.50 on a Saturday morning. Little did they know what they were letting themselves in for! I persuaded Rebecca to come with me and two weeks later we walked into Shappelles dance school in Caerphilly town hall, where the class was full of little girls wearing sparkly Cuban heels. That was where my love affair with dance really began – I fell in love with the shoes. I was desperate for my own pair of Cuban heels.

Our teachers were the former Welsh dance champions Philip and Carol Perry, the most attractive and glamorous couple I'd ever met in my life.

'Do you know what style of dancing we do here?' Philip asked me.

I was ready with my answer. 'Yes, you do Latin, you do American, you do ballroom—'

'Well, that's more or less right,' he said, laughing.

I loved that first class at Shappelles so much that I danced all the way home. I danced around our house all weekend, I danced to school on Monday, and during break I had all my friends dancing in the playground with me.

Two weeks later, Philip Perry called my mum to one side. 'We think Amy's got something you can't teach,' he told her.

Mum raised her eyebrows. 'Well, she doesn't stop dancing, if that's what you mean!'

The Saturday class became the highlight of my week: I'd get so excited that I'd wake up at the crack of dawn and start doing a cha-cha outside my parents' bedroom door. 'Come on, it's time to go!'

'Get back into bed, Amy,' they'd mumble sleepily. 'The class doesn't start for another five hours!'

They couldn't even take me to the supermarket without me dancing down the aisles. People would be dodging their trolleys around this crazy kid doing quickstep and high kicks while they were trying to choose their soup. It was probably best to avoid the supermarket when we did our weekly shop, if I'm honest, because it only took a good song to come on the PA system and I'd be off, making the most of all that space.

Now that I'd found my passion and made this strong connection between movement and music, I constantly wanted to express it. Soon I was learning the basic steps of all the ballroom dances: Latin American, with its samba, rumba, paso doble, cha-cha and jive, and Standard, with the waltz, tango, Viennese waltz, quickstep and foxtrot. And I also did a disco routine that I used to call 'the fuzz'.

At Christmas, Mum and Dad gave me and Rebecca identical red satin Latin dresses made by a neighbour. They had decorative roses on them and the fullest skirts you could imagine – you only had to do a little turn and they lifted and swirled. As I was a super girly girl who loved glitter and pink feather boas, I couldn't have been more thrilled. And my granddad gave us our first pair of Cuban heels – mine were gold and Rebecca's were silver – and I've never loved a pair of shoes as much. I've still got them to this day, tucked away safely at home.

✦

'Would Amy like to join our team at the British Open Formation Championships?' Philip Perry asked my mum, a couple of months after I'd started learning to dance. 'We go to Blackpool every year to compete there, the weekend after

Easter. She'll be in reserve because she's only just joined, but she might like to come along anyway.'

'I'll ask her,' my mum said, but she didn't need to. It was a yes if it was anything to do with dancing, even if it was only in reserve. And, by then, even I knew that Blackpool was the centre of the ballroom and Latin dancing world, where all the important competitions took place and all the best British and international dancers competed.

Formation is a type of competitive ballroom dancing where four or eight couples perform a synchronised routine. It's all about making patterns and staying aligned as a team, and it can be really fun if you're dancing with your friends every week and going off to competitions together. As everyone in the Shappelles formation team was friendly and welcoming to me, I was thrilled to be included in the trip to Blackpool.

We drove up there on the Friday and after Mum and I had checked into our hotel room, she took me to see some of the sights. I'll never forget seeing the famous Blackpool Tower ballroom for the first time: its huge, gleaming dance floor and elegant chandeliers rose up before my eight-year-old eyes like a shimmering dream. It was so impressive that the only thing I could compare it to was Walt Disney World in Florida, where my parents had taken us earlier that year after my beloved nan passed away and left my mum some money.

'Mam, this is better than Disney World!' I said.

Mum chuckled. 'Is it now?'

It was the start of a magical weekend for me. I was dazzled by this wonderland of competitive dancing. As I watched couple after couple whirl across the dance floor, I tried to memorise every new move I saw, every flick of the ankle and wrist, the holds and lifts and pirouettes. And all the while there was one main thought in my mind: *When I grow up, I want to be a professional dancer.*

When it was time to leave, I didn't want to go. Mum had to bribe me away with the promise of sweets.

The world under-12s and under-16s world championships were also taking place that weekend and there were young couples representing countries far and wide – some that I'd never even heard of. Their dancing was so accomplished that it took my breath away and I was amazed to see so many boys among them – Ukrainians, Russians, Americans, you name it – all brilliant dancers. Before *Strictly Come Dancing* exploded onto our screens and gave young boys the confidence to pursue their dreams, there weren't many boys who danced in the UK. It was about 99 per cent girls to 1 per cent boys – and the formation teams in my age group were made up of girls.

'I want one of them boys,' I said to my dance teacher.

He just laughed. I wouldn't be deterred, though. I kept on at him for weeks afterwards. 'Have you got me one of them boys yet?'

There was an English dancer I kept thinking about. He was a few years older than me and I couldn't get over his energy and charisma when he danced – or the spectacular knee slide he'd done halfway through his jive. 'What's his name?' I asked my teacher.

'Him? Kevin Clifton.'

I want to be like him, I thought.

'If you want to get anywhere near his level, you'll have to practise very hard,' my teacher said.

Fortunately, my parents had taught us from an early age that you don't get anything without working for it, and I went for it – with my steps and hold, my rhythm and timing, down to every last detail. I practised. And practised. Every spare minute I had.

Rebecca was my first partner, which was handy for both of us. My sister was a super-talented dancer and loved ballroom with a passion; she also danced in the formation team and did really well. We used to practise at home for hours together, pretending we were at Blackpool competing in the British National Dance Championships, known as the 'Nationals', which are held in November. I probably bossed her around a bit too much, but she didn't mind, although it became clear in time that, for her, dancing was about being with friends and having fun. Whereas, for me, it was my life.

Rebecca and I were born at Caerphilly Miners' Hospital, on 10 August 1990; I arrived first and she came along fifteen minutes later. Right from the start, she was the most chilled person ever – and I was the stress-head. That didn't change as we grew up, either: I was the ultra-competitive sister, the people-pleaser, the one racing to finish my homework first, and probably a bit of a nightmare for her to have around at times. From an early age, I took it upon myself to think for the two of us. I was in charge of our dinner money and if there were letters to give in at school, I'd say, 'I'll take those.' I was the one who came out of primary school one day, stood at the top of the steps and shouted out in front of everyone, 'Rebecca has been in big trouble today! The teacher wrote her name on the board because she was caught talking.'

'Oh, I'd forgotten about that,' Rebecca said, without a care in the world.

I thought I was responsible for her, so I regularly gave her the evil eye in dance class if I thought she was doing something she shouldn't be. I don't know how she put up with it, but I couldn't have had a nicer sister: she always stayed calm; she never retaliated or reacted, except with a smile. My brother, Lloyd, is also really placid and they both still tease me about being the uptight one, especially Rebecca. 'Amy, are you sure you don't want to leave *now*?' she'll say, the night before we're going to the airport, because I get so worried about being late that I'm always super early, to *everything*.

A year after I'd gone to Blackpool as a reserve, I danced there with Rebecca as official members of the formation team – and we won.

'Amy's got what it takes,' my dance teachers told my parents. 'But let's nurture her, let's not push her too soon.'

It was good advice, and we didn't really have a choice, either. Dancing is an expensive sport: it's about lessons, outfits, travel, competitions and studio time, and my parents didn't have the time or money to be driving up and down the country to competitions and lessons every weekend. They devoted their lives to Lloyd, Rebecca and me – they gave us so much support and love – but Dad was already doing freelance carpentry jobs in the evenings and at weekends, on top of his day job as a carpenter at a property development company. He worked so hard to provide for our family. And we all had hobbies, not just me.

Mum encouraged each of us to follow our own individual paths, especially me and Rebecca. She used to say to our teachers Philip and Carol, 'Don't hold one back if you're worried there's not space for both of them in the team. They have to learn. This is life.'

Inevitably, however, we were compared to one another, and as we were always together and shared the same friendship groups, there wasn't much chance to develop our separate identities fully. I think we both started to feel it when we left primary school and moved up to secondary school together, along with the friends we'd had from nursery onwards. It was a great school and Rebecca quickly settled in, and Lloyd was already there and doing well academically, but I wasn't happy, even though I had my friends around me and the teaching was good. It was hugely disappointing for me that dancing wasn't on the school curriculum. There were no school dance facilities, either – what was I even doing in this waste of space?

By this time, Dad had built a back extension and a side extension onto our semi-detached house, so that Rebecca and I could have our own bedrooms, and he laid laminate flooring in the side room, which used to be the playroom, so that we could practise our dancing. There was a piano in there, too, which my brother played brilliantly; Rebecca played the cornet and I played the clarinet for a while. Our poor neighbours had all that going on and on top of it I'd be dancing and stamping around.

But I couldn't practise all the time and within a few days of breaking up from school for the Christmas holiday, I was fidgety and bored. With Shappelles closed for the break, too, what would I do with my days? Rebecca and Lloyd were quite happy to be plonked on the sofa in front of a festive film, but I couldn't even sit down to watch a cartoon all the way through.

My parents treated us to a trip to Winter Wonderland in Cardiff, hoping it would wear me out. It was 23 December, or 'Christmas Eve eve', as I always called it; off we went to Cardiff Castle, buzzing with excitement. But when we got there, my energy seeped away, like air out of a balloon; I turned ghostly white and started feeling unwell. Imagine: you're taking an eleven-year-old kid ice skating, it's Christmas, and suddenly they've got no energy. You *definitely* know something's up. My parents thought I must be coming down with a bug. Then I was sick, so we left.

Back at home, I went straight up to bed, feeling awful. But lying down only seemed to make me feel worse. Then, as I curled up under the covers trying to fight off nausea, I was hit by an excruciating pain in my tummy. I screamed out in agony and my parents came running upstairs. They found me on the bedroom floor, clutching my middle and shrieking.

'What is it, love? What's wrong?' they asked frantically.

I was in that much pain that I couldn't even tell them what was happening. I started being sick again and had a violent attack of diarrhoea.

Terrified that it was appendicitis, my parents rushed me to A&E, where the doctors quickly ran some tests. The results came back negative, which puzzled everyone, and the consultant decided to keep me in overnight, just to be on the safe side.

The next day was Christmas Eve and I felt better, although not brilliant, and I begged the doctors to let me go home.

They ummed and ahed. They were happy with my vital signs, but worried that the excruciating pain might return. While we were discussing what to do, the hospital kitchen staff started bringing dinner round: chicken stew and mashed potato. 'OK, you can go home today, but only if you can eat some dinner first,' the doctors decided.

I looked at my plate in dismay. Hospital food isn't all that great at the best of times, and it's especially unappetising when you've got an upset tummy. 'I can't face it,' I whispered to my parents. 'Dad, will you eat it for me when they're not looking?'

My mum shook her head. 'He can't do that!'

Dad made a face, but he was keen to get me home and it wasn't like the doctors were planning to do surgery on me, or even any tests. It was Christmas, a holding period; nothing was happening in the hospital. He took a deep breath and gobbled up my chicken stew. Bless him!

When I held up my clean plate to the nurses, they let me go, which was a relief. But I started feeling ill again during the discharge process and by the time we got to the hospital entrance I was on the point of collapse. 'Let's take her back,' my mum said anxiously.

'No, please, Mam!' I begged. 'I need to go home. Can you bring the car to the entrance, Dad?'

'No, that won't work,' he said. 'I'll have to carry you.' As he lifted me up, I was sick all down his back.

Somehow they got me home, where my granddad took one look at me and declared, 'She's too ill to be here! She should be in hospital.'

'Please, Gramps,' I said, 'I just want to be with all of you for Christmas.'

For the next few days, I spent a very restless time on the sofa – not in agony, but not really myself. So it wasn't the Christmas I had hoped for, but it was so much better than being in the hospital that I tried not to mind.

We were shaken by what had happened, but were hoping it was a one-off – maybe some kind of blockage in my digestive system that had righted itself. Then I had another attack just a couple of weeks later, and my mum started to suspect that it was Crohn's disease, a chronic condition caused by inflammation in the bowel. We had relatives on both sides of the family who had already been diagnosed with Crohn's.

The doctors dismissed Mum's suggestion that it could be Crohn's, probably because it wasn't such a well-known illness then as it is now. As my health declined in the months to come, they kept telling my parents, 'We don't know what this is.' Perhaps it was hormonal, they said, or a 'grumbling appendix'. Mum started getting frustrated. It was horrific for her and Dad to see their little girl rolling around in agony and being sick, and they naturally wanted answers – or at least a willingness to investigate. But although some of the medical staff were really sympathetic, we seemed to see someone different every time and it never felt like it was the right person. After each appointment, we'd come home none the wiser.

In the absence of any help, Mum wrote a food diary to see if there was any connection between my attacks and certain foods I was eating. That armed us with a tiny bit more knowledge, but without a diagnosis it felt like we were groping around in the dark.

'Nobody knows your daughter like you do,' advised my mum's auntie, who was a medical lecturer. 'You're the one who knows when something isn't right, and if you're not happy, you've got to keep on pushing.'

Mum often stayed overnight in the hospital with me, which was hard because she had two children at home as well. As a child, you don't realise the toll it takes on your parents to sit on a chair all night by your bed, but it must have been exhausting. She had to take loads of time off work, too, which added to the strain. And still the doctors didn't seem to be listening.

'This isn't my little girl,' she used to tell them, as I lay lifeless on the hospital bed, too poorly to get up and go to the toilet. 'This isn't the Amy who bounces around the living room and drives us up the wall because we can't even watch a soap with her there. She's like a bottle of pop normally.'

I was in hospital that many times over the next couple of years that I lost count. Dad spent endless long hours at the hospital as well, keeping me company while Mum was running around and trying to get answers.

'I'd do anything to take this pain away from you,' he'd say, as he stroked my forehead and held my hand. 'I wish it was me, not you.'

For someone as active and sporty as me, it was a nightmare being forced to rest every time I got ill. I dealt with it by staying busy in my mind, constantly working out dance moves and imagining how life would be if I could dance as much as I wanted to. You've always got to hold on to hope and I tried to stay positive; fortunately, I'm the kind of person who sees the glass as being half full, rather than half empty, and I try to see the good in everything – in people and scenarios.

But in my low moments, my dancing dreams sometimes seemed to be nothing more than that – just dreams. I felt it especially when family and friends came to visit, because they weren't asking me about my dancing any more. Instead it was, 'How's your health? How's your tummy?' I wished they would just ask me, 'How's your dancing?' I wanted to be known as 'Amy the dancer', not 'Amy with the mysterious illness that we suspect is Crohn's'.

'You'll have to stop dancing now, I suppose,' people said, their eyes full of sympathy.

'No, I won't. I'm fine most of the time,' I used to say defensively.

If anything, being poorly made me want to dance more, not less, because it was all I thought about when I was recovering. I'm a goal-driven person and I like to have something to look forward to, so I found it helped when I imagined what I'd be learning in my next dance class.

'But maybe you need to take it easy for a while,' people kept on telling me.

I knew they were speaking from a place of kindness, but they didn't seem to understand that missing out on a dance class for me was worse than waking up on my birthday with no presents. And the suggestion that my dancing could be taken away altogether put my teeth on edge. I was absolutely determined to keep going and improving.

So I'd smile and pretend they hadn't rubbed me up the wrong way. 'Actually, I can't wait to start dancing again,' I'd tell them, and they'd shrug, as if to say, 'On your own head be it.'

I'll admit they had a point about taking it easy, though, because I pushed myself too hard and started dancing too soon. It was impossible to resist going into the dance studio once I was up and about. I desperately wanted to be like the other children and get back to doing what I loved. I never liked the feeling of giving up.

Why me? Why am I always ill? I'd think in frustration. And why doesn't anybody know what's wrong with me?

I didn't dwell on it, though, because what's the point of sitting around and complaining? Life was teaching me to pick myself up when I fell down, to dust myself off and keep going. As soon as I was well again, I practised harder than ever.

Chapter 2

Fail to prepare, prepare to fail

Dancing was everything to me. It made me feel free and happy, and I had a constant drive to improve, so it was devastating that my progress was stalled every time I got sick. But the way I saw it, I'd never had anything given to me on a plate – I'd had to work hard for everything and make my own chances. Sometimes things came good and sometimes they didn't. And the only way to succeed was to keep trying.

So when someone told me that there were performing arts schools in London where you could study dance and drama as part of the curriculum, I decided to find out more. *Why can't I go to one of those schools?* I thought, picturing how amazing it would be to immerse myself in the world of dance, to have lessons every day and guidance from top teachers.

I did some research towards the end of Year Seven and found out that some of the schools offered scholarships and bursaries to promising students. Would I have any chance of getting one? Why not try anyway?

So, without my mum and dad knowing – just because I wasn't sure how they would react – I started sending off applications for scholarships at performing arts schools.

Suddenly, my parents were getting all these brochures and

prospectuses through the post, and it didn't take a genius to guess what was going on. 'You're not moving to London, Amy,' they said.

'But I just want to dance!' I told them. 'At these schools you can do seventy per cent dance and thirty per cent academic subjects.'

'You're far too young to start living in London without your mum and dad,' Mum replied. 'And what would you do if you got sick while you were down there and we couldn't get to you?'

She was right that I needed to stay at home, safe in my family cocoon, but I hated being held back by something I couldn't control. I guess I learned a lesson, though: however big your dreams are, you need to be realistic about how you're going to achieve them. As there was no way Mum and Dad were going to let me go and live in London – and they couldn't drive me around the country for expensive private lessons or competitions, either – I had to find another way to keep my dancing dreams alive.

Then my luck changed, as luck always does. 'Amy, guess what?' a friend said to me one day, towards the end of the year. 'Have you heard of a school called St Cenydd? They're building a new leisure centre facility and it's got a dance studio inside it.'

My heart skipped a beat. Was she winding me up?

'Amy, you're a dancer – you should go there!' she went on. 'There's a dance department and a dance teacher. You can do GCSE dance there.'

'You are joking!' I screeched. I couldn't wait to get home and tell my parents.

Mum and Dad didn't exactly leap at the idea, though. 'A new school? But it's miles outside our catchment area. And even if you got a place there, you wouldn't know anyone. You'd be leaving all your friends behind.'

'But, Mum, they've got a dance studio! And I can see my friends at the weekend.'

There were other considerations, though. What about the illness that kept stopping me in my tracks? How would I cope if I had an attack while I was still settling into my new school? And perhaps I shouldn't put all my eggs in one basket. Yes, dancing made me happy, but I was good academically, too. Maybe I should put my studies first. And the school I was already in was great in lots of other ways ...

There was also the cost of a new school uniform to take into account, and the daily bus fare to and from St Cenydd. My mum and dad worked hard and we'd been taught to understand and appreciate the value of money, so I didn't like the idea of adding to their bills. But at the same time I desperately wanted to go to this school – I *needed* to go to this school.

'I'll earn my own bus fare! Carol says I can start teaching at Shappelles when I'm thirteen ...' I said, and listed every moneymaking idea I could think of.

I argued, I pleaded, I begged, I wheedled – and every time my parents came up with a reason against going to St Cenydd, I'd say something like, 'But you were the ones who told me to always believe in myself!' and, 'You taught me to be determined and to go after my goals in life!'

Eventually I persuaded them to get in contact with both the local council and the school, to see if there was a way of getting me a place there. Phone calls were made, forms filled in, letters posted, and at last I was invited to go and have a look around. Now it was down to me to convey my love and passion for dancing to the deputy head and head teacher, and I think I did quite a good job of it, because they agreed to take me – in theory. Only, the school was full, they said, and they didn't have a place for me.

It was a huge disappointment and I tried not to plunge into gloom and despair. Instead, I spent the whole summer holidays on alert, hoping for a miracle. Every day I checked the mail to see if there was a letter from St Cenydd saying, 'Yes, Amy can come!' Every time the landline rang, I wondered if this was the moment I'd be jumping for joy. I tried as hard as I could to believe that whatever the outcome, things would work out for the best. I practised and practised my dancing.

Two days before the autumn term started, my wish finally came true. And so, on my first day of Year Eight, instead of walking to school with Rebecca and joining up with friends along the way, I headed alone into the town centre and got on the bus to St Cenydd.

It was only a ten-minute bus ride, but it felt like independence, and I was thrilled that my determination had paid off. But I don't think I was prepared for how scary it is to walk into a new school where I knew absolutely nobody. There's all this hustle and bustle around you, and people screaming their hellos after the long summer break – you feel about as significant as a flea under a blanket.

While I tried to settle in, I had moments of thinking, *Have I done the right thing?* Would I be better off back in my comfort zone with my sister and friends? But as soon as I started the dance lessons, I liked the dance teacher, Rhianwen Moore, which helped. She had trained with Philip and Carol when she was growing up, and although we didn't do much ballroom in her classes, we learned a bit of everything, from contemporary dance to ballet and musical theatre. And Miss Moore always believed in me as a dancer and was always ready to help me with my flexibility, or to stay on late at school so that I could practise in the studio. At the same time, I was starting to build a group of good friends and find my place, so I began to think that, yes, it was the right decision to move to St Cenydd.

It actually turned out to be a positive move in many ways. Rebecca and I had been by one another's side since the day we were born, but now that we weren't being lumped together as 'the twins', we were able to develop our own separate identities. Nobody at my new school even knew I had a twin sister, so there was no comparing, and that was definitely a good thing – for both of us individually, and for our relationship. We'd taken to bickering a bit in Year Seven, but now, when we met up at home after being apart all day, we were happy to see each other and couldn't wait to share what we'd been up to at school. Mind you, I still wanted to beat her at anything and everything – and she still wasn't bothered. She was doing incredibly well at school and had a big group of friends, so she was happy.

We went on dancing together, until eventually I think even she found me a bit too bossy and competitive to partner with. I was a perfectionist and drove myself hard; I wanted to practise all the time, and Rebecca would say, 'No, I'm watching a cartoon now.'

But I wouldn't give up; I would nag and nag. 'She's holding me back!' I'd complain, and my parents realised that this wasn't going to work.

Maybe that's why Philip and Carol thought I had what it takes to be a dancer. I was totally committed and didn't want to miss a single opportunity to dance, whereas Rebecca was very much into everything – from football, tennis and skateboarding, to playing the piano (which we both did) – and she also played the cornet in the school orchestra.

Aged twelve, I finally got a male dance partner; his name was Gino Gabriela, he was dark-haired with sparkling blue eyes, and he was practically the only boy in Caerphilly who didn't have two left feet, as far as I could tell. I was thrilled to pair up with Gino, and not only because he was a boy: he was a great dancer and a lot of fun. Gino became a fixture at our house and my parents welcomed him in, partly because he kept me occupied and tired me out, I think – he was the perfect friend for me, in their eyes! And Rebecca started dancing with her best friend from school, so it all worked out perfectly.

✦

In the summer of 2004, when I didn't think I could be any more obsessed with dancing, *Strictly Come Dancing* hit our screens for the first time. I was nearly fourteen years old and everything about the show entranced me. I had never seen anything so wonderful in my life; I was absolutely in awe of all the professionals, their dresses and the way they danced. When Season 2 got under way later that year, I started to live for Saturday nights from September to Christmas, and every Sunday me and my granddad would critique the dances and try to guess who'd be voted out. By now, I was telling everybody, 'I want to be a professional dancer on *Strictly Come Dancing*.'

'Yeah, wouldn't that be nice?' people said. 'But those dancers have all reached the top and won pro championship titles and trophies. It's a different world, Amy.'

I knew what they were thinking: that it was an impossible dream for a small-town girl like me who kept collapsing and having to go to hospital. But *Strictly* was a massive inspiration – for me and my sister, Rebecca. We would tape it and play it back over and over after school: I'd be dancing for her and getting her to give me scores; if we saw any tricky or clever choreography, we'd practise it until we thought we'd got it right. *Strictly* filled my head with dreams – of dancing, sequinned costumes, glitter balls and glamour. It kept me going every time I had another attack of suspected Crohn's disease.

Now that *Strictly Come Dancing* was lighting up my life, my drive to dance rocketed even higher, if that was possible. I had to take a break from couples dancing when Gino moved out of the area for a while, but I was still busy with the formation team. I also started doing ballet and put a lot of work into it, knowing it would help my dancing training; I got to grade six and began doing pointe work, which I absolutely loved. I wanted to be in the studio at school every single day if they'd let me; every morning I'd go in early and be knocking at the dance teacher's door, saying, 'Can I go up yet?' I stayed after school for dance clubs; I went on to study performing arts.

The school pushed and supported me, even as they

witnessed my health battles and all the setbacks I faced trying to get better from my illness. Some of the staff started to recognise the signs that I was about to have an attack – I guess it wasn't that hard to see when something was wrong, because I was usually a conscientious and energetic student who loved being in school and who worked hard, and then suddenly I'd have no life about me. Everything would be a struggle. My eyes would swell up, which was a warning sign that I was getting ill, and the school would ring my mum, saying, 'Amy's eyes are swollen. Can you come and get her?'

I used to hate having time off: I was constantly worried that I'd fall behind in class and my results would suffer. So I'd carry on until the very last minute, dragging myself around, pretending nothing was wrong. Then the pain would come on so fast – it would literally strike me like a knife in the gut, and sometimes it was so intense that I passed out. It was scary for my friends and the other kids at school to see a fellow student carted off on a stretcher and screaming her head off. I think the head teacher and the staff found it really worrying, too. For me, it was highly embarrassing, because I felt so out of control, and as I still hadn't been diagnosed, how could I explain it to anyone?

My teachers didn't ease up on me, though. They didn't make allowances for my health, because they knew how determined I was to do the best I could. I guess I was one of those characters: even if I wasn't top at everything, I'd only ever want to give 100 per cent. Dancing was my number one priority, so if I didn't get full marks and the teacher only gave me, say, 29 out of 30, I'd be thinking, *Why did I lose that last mark?* And it wasn't just dancing, it was everything. If I was aiming for a B in History and I got a C, I'd be knocking on the teacher's door, asking, 'So what do I have to do to get a B?' It makes me sound like I was trying to be a teacher's pet, but it wasn't that. We're hard workers in our family – it's the way we were raised – and I had this burning desire to do well.

The whole time I was at school, there was a banner up in the assembly hall emblazoned with the motto, 'Fail to prepare, prepare to fail.' I took it to heart and some of the teachers found me a bit exasperating, I think. My old PE teacher recently reminded me of the many times I burst into his office to ask a question, almost always just as he was sitting down during the lunch break to eat his nice cooked dinner.

There'd be a knock at the door and it would be Amy 'can-I-use-the-dance-studio' Dowden saying, 'I've got a question.'

Knife and fork in hand, teeth gritted, he'd ask, 'Do you need to know the answer right now?'

'Well, yes, if you don't mind.'

It would never be a straightforward question that he could answer on the spot and get back to his dinner, he says. He'd have to get the textbook, because I needed to know everything in great detail. And all the while he'd be aware that his nice hot dinner was cooling down and congealing.

I'm grateful that when I was growing up I had people who I could look up to, who pushed themselves and never took things for granted. My granddad had worked all hours to build his own business from scratch. My father worked seven days a week sometimes, and evenings. My brother, Lloyd, studied hard and worked at Kwik Save both at the weekend and on two weekday evenings throughout sixth form and university. They were all great role models. They taught me that you have to work hard in order to get what you want.

Lloyd never complained about the noise I made while I was practising, either. Someone would say, 'Where's Lloyd?' and we'd find him sitting in his Micra car, studying in peace, instead of telling me to turn the music down. Then he'd come back in when I started on my homework. Because, of course, I took my cue from him and never missed doing my homework.

I also had a business side that started to come out. My friends used to ask in assembly, 'Ames, have you done your maths? Can I copy?' I always said yes, and when I got older, I'd say, 'Yes, for fifty pence!' or, 'Yes, if you share your sandwich with me.' Sometimes I'd sell the sandwiches in my packed lunch and put the money towards the fake eyelashes or fake tan I needed for my dancing competitions. But that enterprise came to an end when one of the boys said to my mum, 'Do you think you could put butter in Amy's sandwiches, please?'

'Why?' Mum said, knowing I didn't like butter.

'I buy them off Amy!'

✦

I was fifteen when Gino moved back into the area and we started dancing as a couple again. We were so happy to be spending time with each other again that we practised harder than ever, and soon we were entering competitions all around Wales. Carol and Philip supported us all the way: they helped fund our lessons so that we could dance together and gave us free time in the studio to practise; they did everything they could to help us to progress and achieve. I owe them so much.

Gino was only dancing for fun, really, but I used to make him do hours of extra practice when we had a competition coming up. 'Right, we're up at six tomorrow morning to work on our jive before we go!' I'd insist.

He could see my drive and determination, and always believed I could go all the way. 'When Amy gets married, she'll be on the front of *Hello!* magazine!' he used to say.

We just laughed at him. 'Don't be so silly!'

These days, my mum sometimes gets the same bus as him on the way into work in the mornings. 'I told you, didn't I, Gill?' he says to her.

Gino and I started doing well in the Welsh competitions. We even won the Welsh Open Championships when we were seventeen. That was exciting – Colin Jackson, the TV presenter and former athlete, and a BBC Wales film crew followed our journey. But it was one thing winning titles in Wales and something else altogether to make our mark in England, where we were often up against dancers who came from wealth, or whose parents were judges or champion pro dancers. (I call it pedigree!) These were kids who could afford to have dance lessons whenever they wanted, or to buy a new costume and new shoes before every competition. What chance did we have against them, with our one hour of tuition a week? Our dance lessons at school helped with movement and rhythm, but what we really needed was more focused Latin American dance training.

Most of the time we didn't make it beyond the first round, but we didn't let it bother us. We just loved the atmosphere of the big competitions and being around the top dancers. I guess there was a part of me that wanted to be one of the top girls dancing with the top boys, though. To wear the best dresses and go up and down the country having lessons with famous coaches. To be someone who the judges knew by name, and who automatically made it through to the finals. I could see how good they were and my parents could, too.

How am I going to get that good? I'd think, mesmerised by their incredible dancing and beautiful dresses. Teachers and professionals used to come up to me and Gino, and say how talented we were and ask where we were from, but although in Wales I was fast becoming a big fish in a small pond, in England I was a nobody.

Never mind, I thought, *I'll just work harder.*

And when I look back I think it was probably good for me that I was only doing small competitions, because I never had the chance to burn myself out, as some dancers did.

✦

Dancing is so expensive that, as soon as I was able, I started earning money to pay for extra lessons and costumes. The year before my A levels, as well as waitressing in a pizza restaurant and teaching at a dance studio, I worked the whole summer in a hair salon (£1.20 an hour, apprentice wage!) to buy myself a flesh-and-pink dance dress, covered in diamantés. I can't tell you how much I loved that dress. I didn't take anything for granted now: as I was handing over the cash for each dance lesson, knowing how hard I'd worked to get it, I was determined to make the most of the class and absorb every nugget of learning. That summer, Gino and I practised really hard, either at the school dance studio or at Philip and Carol's. We only danced Latin together – lots of high-energy cha-chas and paso dobles, and, as I was always pushing us the extra mile, we steadily improved.

Later in the year, Dad took us to the UK under-21s Latin American championships in Bournemouth. We weren't expecting to get far – we were literally the only couple in that competition who were going in with one session of private tuition a week – although we couldn't help hoping, of course. But really we were there for the experience rather than the results, because everything about it was so exciting. We also went to Blackpool after Easter every year and danced in the British Open Formation Championships for the fun of it – even though back then couple dancers didn't do formation dancing, as the styles are very different. I loved formation – there was always a great team spirit and it taught me discipline – but the level of competition in couples dancing is much tougher and I wanted that next challenge.

When we made it to the semi-finals at the championships in Bournemouth we were absolutely thrilled. It was a total 'wow' moment and we couldn't stop grinning. Dad was over the moon, too. He went off to the bar to buy a celebratory drink.

We felt we danced well in the semi-finals, but you can never really tell how you've done in ballroom dancing, because your result depends on the opinion of the judges. It's not like crossing the finishing line as an athlete, when you've either won or you haven't. So when the final was announced and our numbers were called, we looked at each other in utter amazement. My dad was so surprised that he dropped his pint.

We jumped for joy and ran onto the dance floor. I could

sense the crowd bristling with curiosity. People were think-ing, *Who are they?*

There was no way we were going to win – first and second places in the final went to the children of professional ball-room dancers, as you'd expect. Still, we couldn't believe it when we came sixth out of everyone. It was an amaz-ing achievement. And almost the best thing about it was seeing how proud Carol and Philip were of us afterwards. We couldn't have been more grateful to them, because we would never have got that result without their generosity and encouragement.

That day I had a realisation: *Yes, I can do this! This is where I belong, in the ballroom and Latin world. If I can make it to the final with so little extra coaching, then imagine what I could do with the right partner, lessons and training.*

✦

I felt torn, even though it was clear that Gino and I were heading in different directions: I lived for dance, but for Gino it was a hobby; his goal was to go into hairdressing and open his own salon, whereas I wanted to make it as a Latin American dancer. But a big part of me didn't want to say goodbye to my lovely friend, who had always been supportive when I was ill. He never complained when we were forced to have a week off training or weren't able to compete. Once he'd stayed with me all night after I had a sudden attack during a competition in Worcester and ended up in hospital. And Gino and I had so much fun together, too. So it was hard to split, although thankfully, when it finally happened, we stayed good friends. He still dances beautifully to this day.

Now I needed to find a boy I could go to the next level with, but the boy–girl imbalance meant that the boys had the pick of the girls, so it was a fiercely competitive process. I was looking for someone who was the right height at about five feet ten inches, well known and had good results in competition – better results than mine, if I'm honest – which narrowed the field. And although I was hoping that my health issues wouldn't hold me back or put anybody off, I'm sure they did.

When a boy became available, he usually advertised himself on the dance websites or in the weekly dance newspaper. Or sometimes Philip or Carol would ring me and say they'd heard of someone suitable and I'd contact his teacher or mum to suggest setting up a dance tryout. I'd often go along hoping this was the one: I'd make sure that I looked as pretty as I could and had my best dress on; I'd be really smiley and chatty and give it my all. My heart would soar when his teacher nodded approvingly and said, 'Yes, interested.' Only for it to break when they called afterwards and said, 'We're really sorry, we've gone for another girl.'

I knew when I was trying out with certain boys that they weren't picking me because of my health. As soon as some of my potential partners – or their teachers – heard about my illness on the dance circuit, they didn't want to know. It felt very unfair: it would have been easier to accept if I'd been rejected because I lived too far away, or needed to improve my ballroom dancing. But it wasn't because my dancing wasn't good enough – it was because of something I couldn't control or change.

'It's not my fault,' I'd say to Carol. 'I didn't ask to have all these tummy problems.'

Carol and Philip went above and beyond to help me. Philip was confident I had what it takes to get to the top, so he never stopped encouraging me to go for a dance career, even when everyone else was against it because of my illness. Carol was also very supportive: she would give me teaching jobs so that I could pay for extra lessons; she would drive me to competitions, or to Birmingham for tryouts with boys, and let me train for free in the studio. I was lucky to have these amazing angels in my life. They're like a second mum and dad to me, and I'm like the daughter they never had.

They couldn't help worrying about me, though. Seeing me collapse on the dance studio floor and get rushed off in an ambulance made them hesitant about putting too much pressure on me and causing me stress. There were times when Carol wouldn't want me to dance, because she was so concerned I was going to make myself worse. But, being a dancer herself, she understood that I just wanted to push on.

I kept going to tryouts; I kept being knocked back. You have to be resilient when you're a dancer. You can't always dance your best; you can't win every competition – I had to accept that rejection is part of the journey. I refused to give up.

There is going to be somebody out there who will dance with me and understand, I kept telling myself.

✦

In the months leading up to my A levels, my parents understandably tried to steer me towards education and studying. For them, the safe and stable option was to go to university and study English, which would set me up for a solid future in teaching, or another profession. As my illness wasn't getting any better, they felt that a profession like teaching would be a lot more forgiving than a career in dancing.

I didn't know what to do. I knew I'd enjoy going to uni, because I loved learning and working hard. I was that student who did so much revision for my A levels that there wasn't enough room on the exam papers for me to write everything I'd learned, the one who scribbled down every relevant piece of information that was in my brain until I ran out of space and had to use the margins. That was me. All or nothing.

I also couldn't forget how poorly I'd been in the past year. Triggered by the stress and pressure of impending A levels, my illness had come back with a vengeance and I was in horrific pain during a couple of my exams: I was sweating buckets and going back and forth to the bathroom, literally passing black tar, during one of my English papers.

I applied for a place on a degree course at a dance school in London, which would give me the tools and qualification to be a dance teacher. It was a fantastic place, a creative hub bang in the centre of London with amazing facilities and teachers. The problem was that it was a contemporary dance degree and I wouldn't be able to continue with my Latin and ballroom dancing. So although I was thrilled when they offered me a scholarship at my audition, it put me in a dilemma.

I remember the day I made my mind up once and for all. It was the day I went to pick up my A level results at school – three As and a C.

The local newspaper in Caerphilly wanted to do an interview because I'd done so well. 'So which university are you going to?' the reporter asked, looking impressed.

Suddenly it came to me. Yes, dancing was a precarious career. But I was hardworking and determined. I had experienced tough times and disappointments. I knew how to bounce back from pain and injury.

In just a few years, life had taught me extreme resilience. And anyway, sometimes you just have to go with your instinct, don't you?

'Oh no, I'm not going to uni,' I told the reporter. 'I'm gonna go and fulfil my dancing dreams.'

His face fell. 'What?' He clearly thought I was crazy. I could see in his expression what so many people had said to me, 'You'll never make it as a professional dancer. What are you thinking?'

As he shook his head in disbelief at my stupidity, I couldn't help giggling. I could hardly believe that I'd actually come out with it myself. But there was no going back on it now. It was official. I'd told the press!

Chapter 3

You learn more from the downs than the ups

I can't think how many times I've been in hospital. It's got to be over a hundred. For eight years, I was in and out every few months, and no one could say what was wrong with me. It was at its worst when I was between the ages of eighteen and nineteen, and I'd find myself on a ward every month at least, often stuck there for a week or longer. Hospital was like my second home.

I never knew when the next attack of my illness was coming. Mum used to mark it on the calendar: sometimes I'd have a few weeks of being well, sometimes a few months; I was always hoping it had settled down or even gone forever. But then it would flare up again and I'd be back in an ambulance.

Each time it followed a pattern. The pain would come on suddenly. I'd be rushed to hospital screaming in agony. Next came constant vomiting and diarrhoea. Painkillers and anti-nausea medicine would bring me through the worst. And then I'd have to lie in a hospital bed for days on end, getting my strength back.

I met loads of kind, wonderful people during my stays on the ward. But when you're eighteen, you feel that this is your time to go out and explore the world, to become yourself and achieve your dreams, so I hated being stuck in hospital. My sister was at university, living her best life; my brother had graduated and was now doing his master's degree; and there I was, staring at four hospital walls.

✦

My parents could see how ill I was and they were sure it was Crohn's disease, but the doctors were still saying they didn't know what the problem was. Crohn's was not very well known and still underdiagnosed in those days, and I felt as if I was living in limbo, waiting for a breakthrough – the chance to be free of illness. In the meantime, I lived in fear that what I loved the most could be taken away from me.

You learn more from the bad times than the good, I think. Even when I was in hospital with nothing to do, I was learning something. My perception of time changed completely. When you're eighteen and out there living your life, you think you've got all the time in the world. But when you're lying in a hospital bed for days on end, it feels like your life is passing you by. Each day feels like something precious you've lost.

It's like you're in two different zones, though – fast and slow – because as much as the weeks were flying by in the real world, the hours passed so slowly as I lay in my hospital bed that it sometimes felt as if time was at a standstill. The hands on the wall clock didn't even seem to be moving: I'd look up and be stunned that only three minutes had passed since I'd last checked, because it felt like three hours. It was the worst kind of torture when I was waiting for my next set of pain medication: as the morphine wore off and the agony returned, I waited in slow-ticking torment for a nurse to bring my next dose.

Years later, when I was partnered on *Strictly Come Dancing* with the ex-Royal Marine JJ Chalmers, he described going through something similar when he was in rehab after being injured in a bomb blast in Afghanistan. There, time dragged so much that in the end he asked a nurse to take the clock off the wall, and I think I'd do the same if I ever had another long hospital stay. You're better off without it.

I made a promise to myself during those long days on the ward: when I'm well again, I'm going to make the most of every opportunity that comes along; I'm going to push myself, work harder at my dancing and make my dreams come true. And I will never again take being well for granted.

In the meantime, I was desperate for the doctors to decide what was wrong with me so that I could get access to the treatment I needed. My symptoms were typical of Crohn's disease, which causes inflammation and soreness in the gut, the long winding tube that starts at the mouth, travels through the oesophagus, stomach and the small and large intestines, and ends at the anus. Crohn's can lead to diarrhoea, sickness, intense stomach pain, swollen eyes and listlessness, among other things, and I had all of these. But I was getting nowhere near an accurate diagnosis.

Part of the problem was that too little was known about Crohn's disease for many doctors to feel confident in identifying it. My cousins had struggled to get diagnosed with their Crohn's, so I knew I wasn't the only one. It's still not fully understood why someone develops it or how to treat it; why a flare-up happens and when the next is going to come.

One difficulty is that it can affect any part of the intestines, which are at least fifteen feet long. Another is that testing for Crohn's is painful and invasive, so doctors are often reluctant to put a child or a young person through it.

'You clearly don't appreciate the pain she goes through when she has a flare-up,' my mum said. 'No test could be worse than that.'

We had a real problem in being heard by the doctors. A lot of them just weren't listening to what we were saying. Often they didn't see me until the worst of my pain had subsided and then they just saw a poorly girl. The tests they did weren't showing anything – none of the markers were coming up to indicate Crohn's – and maybe they ran out of ideas because of this, so they started suggesting that I had an eating disorder. This was based on no evidence other than that I was slim, and the assumption that as a dancer I'd be watching my weight.

'She just needs to go home and eat a Mars bar,' one doctor said dismissively to my mum. Then he walked off before either of us could reply.

How unfeeling can you be? We were both in tears afterwards. As weight loss is a symptom of Crohn's disease, and I was sick and had diarrhoea every time I was poorly, it made no sense to jump to that conclusion.

'I love my food! But when I'm poorly, I lose my appetite,' I remember saying.

'So you sometimes skip meals?'

'Only when I'm poorly.'

'So you admit to skipping meals when you're not hungry ... You should always eat at mealtimes, you know.'

'Not if I'm going to vomit it straight up again, surely?'

'Do you sometimes make yourself sick deliberately?'

'No! Why would I do that? I want to feel well and be able to dance.'

✦

We just kept going round and round in circles. At one point we even had the feeling they thought I was making everything up – that I was trying to prove I was ill by starving myself, or something crazy like that. 'Is she unhappy at school?' they'd ask.

'No, she genuinely loves going to school,' my parents would say in exasperation.

It didn't make sense to think a normally happy and active kid would choose to be stuck in a hospital bed, when they could be having a nice time with their friends and family, or dancing. But that's what we were dealing with, and it was upsetting and confusing.

Eventually, my mum said, 'If you think she's got anorexia, you should be treating her for that, then, shouldn't you?'

I was so lucky to have my parents fighting my corner! If you have a serious health problem and you feel you're not being listened to or believed by health professionals, you need an advocate like my mum. It's good to know that there are now several charities offering independent advocacy to hospital patients, so if you've got a complaint, or you're having trouble getting your message across, you can ask about finding someone. (I've included a few resources at the back of this book if you need that help.) I can't imagine how much worse things would have been for me if I hadn't had Mum and Dad putting pressure on the doctors on my behalf. How, as a teenager, are you going to cope if doctors say that the illness that is devastating your body is in fact all in your head?

'I'm this shape partly because I'm a dancer and do a lot of exercise,' I'd tell the doctors.

'Well, you'll have to stop dancing,' I was told. 'A career as a professional dancer? Unlikely, I'm afraid.'

How do you know? I'd think. *You may be a doctor but you're not living in my body, with my pain, are you?*

Why did they say it? Just to make me feel worse? That's not what doctors are supposed to do. It helped me in a way, though. It gave me the grit and strength of will to go on, the fire in my belly. I was determined to prove them wrong. *I'll show you*, I'd think. *How dare you? You have no idea.*

It's that 'can't' word that always gets me. It makes me want to explode and shout, 'Yes, I can!' Even today, I have people telling me that my cancer will limit me in a particular way, that I'll suffer this or that, like they did, so I won't be able to dance again or have kids myself. And I try not to listen. We are all individuals. Every journey is different. I'm on my own path, so maybe 'you won't' and 'you can't', but I can and I will.

A chance to diagnose my Crohn's was missed when I was seventeen and had my appendix out. When I came round from surgery, the doctors said they had found a lot of pus around my bowels, which the consultant I have now says was probably a sign of Crohn's disease in my appendix, as my Crohn's is in the terminal ileum, which is attached to the appendix. But I was not referred to a gastroenterologist, who would probably have been able to help more. We didn't give up, though. We started pushing to see an expert in Crohn's. Still nothing happened.

A year after the appendectomy, things became really bad. Almost overnight, I went from having extreme diarrhoea to severe constipation, which may have been a consequence of the doctors giving me medicine for years on end to bung me up and stop me going to the toilet. Now I was so constipated that my gut was backed up and I couldn't keep anything down when I ate. I was constantly being sick and I threw up faecal vomit, which is a sign of bowel obstruction. I smelled really bad; even my skin started smelling of poo, like it was seeping out of my pores. It was repulsive. It would have been tough for anyone, but it was the pits for a really girly girl like me, who loved looking and smelling nice. I felt disgusting.

We now know that my Crohn's disease had narrowed the bowel to the extent that nothing could get through. But at the time we were clueless and I was having to go into hospital for an enema to clear me out every two weeks or so. That changed when, after one appointment, a nurse handed me a plastic bag. 'Here's a do-it-yourself irrigation kit and a how-to DVD, so that you can give yourself enemas at home,' he said, as if he was doing me a favour. 'It'll save you coming here every two weeks.'

It would save a lot of hassle, for sure. I wasn't sure I felt competent, though. 'But how will I know what to do?' I asked.

'There are step-by-step instructions on the DVD. It's all perfectly clear. You'll soon learn.'

'O-kaay, could someone give me a quick demo before I go?'

'No need! It's all there on the DVD,' he said breezily.

I still felt uneasy about it, but he seemed confident it would be fine. Little did I know that if I hadn't done it correctly, I could easily have perforated my bowel and given myself a life-threatening injury, maybe even died as a result. Fortunately, I was careful – or maybe just lucky – and for the next year I didn't have to use my bowel at all because the irrigation kit was doing it for me.

As the attacks of stomach pain and nausea became more frequent, I started to worry more and more about my health. I reached my lowest point when I'd just turned nineteen and was taken to hospital in such agony that I was begging the doctors to slice me open and cut my stomach out. I'd tried to take each attack of my illness in my stride until then, reminding myself that I always made it through and got well again. But now, for the first time, I wasn't so sure. They kept me in the ward for about ten days and the pain wouldn't go away.

My sister, away at university, found it very hard not knowing what was going on. It was terrible for the whole family, but she really went through it, especially when she heard that the surgeons were thinking they might have to take out my colon. She was so worried that she lay awake all night with anxiety pains in her own stomach.

I reached breaking point one night at about four in the morning. I'd taken all the morphine I was allowed to take and the maximum dose of anti-sickness medicine, too, but the pain in my tummy was so unbearable that I felt I just couldn't fight it any more.

With trembling hands, I picked up my phone to call my parents. Just at that moment, I caught the eye of the woman in the opposite bed. Seeing that I was so weak from pain and nausea that I could hardly lift my head from the pillow to speak to them, she heaved herself out of bed and came over to try to help me.

Mum answered the call. 'Amy? What is it, love?'

The tears were pouring down my cheeks; I was strung out with pain. 'I can't do this any more,' I sobbed. 'I just want to go.'

The woman from the opposite bed gently took the phone from me. 'You should come. Your daughter is so, so poorly,' she told my mum.

Mum and Dad raced to the hospital and sat beside me until morning. The following day, Dad rang my consultant and eventually the consultant rang him back. 'We've done every test possible, but they're all inconclusive,' he told Dad.

'It's not good enough. You could do better,' Dad insisted. 'If it was your daughter, she would have got a diagnosis long ago. It would never have gone this far.'

'If it was my daughter, I would be doing exactly the same,' the consultant said.

'No, you wouldn't. You wouldn't have sat back and watched your daughter in so much pain without even knowing what the problem was. By now, you would have said, 'I'm not capable of finding out what it is and I'll find someone who can.' You would do it for your daughter and I want you to do the same for mine.'

One of my aunts who is a nurse had advised Dad to gather evidence to prove the doctors weren't doing enough for me, and by now Dad had filled a thick folder with notes and photocopies. 'Enough is enough,' he told the consultant. He wasn't being rude, but he was probably getting a bit emotional by then. 'If you don't do something to help Amy right now, we're probably going to seek legal advice.'

The consultant decided that he was going to refer me to a top consultant gastroenterologist in London. I was glad that something was finally happening, but at the same time felt frustrated that my life was still on hold until we went to London and I couldn't plan anything.

Since the summer of my A levels, I'd been working full-time in the Cardiff office of Barratt Homes, the company my dad worked for as a carpenter. I worked hard and was always up for doing extra work when I'd finished what I had to do. I used to bargain with the directors: 'Yes, I'll file those papers for you, or take some minutes – if you buy me three bars of chocolate from the vending machine!'

I remember always being hungry while I was working there. One day, I took the minutes for a meeting in the man-aging director's office and couldn't help eyeing up the bowl of biscuits in the middle of the table. I didn't take one during the meeting but when everyone had left, I quickly picked one up and put the whole thing in my mouth. When I turned around, cheeks bulging, there was the managing director! He picked up the bowl of biscuits with a smile and said, 'Would you like one, Amy?'

Whenever I had to go into his office, he knew I was coming because he'd hear a rustling of wrappers as I dipped into the bowl of mints he had outside. He was a great boss and very understanding when I took time off because I was ill. Eventually, I handed in my notice, though, as it wasn't fair on them to be off sick so much.

In the middle of all of this, I went for a tryout with a boy called Tom Parkes, a known dancer. I really liked Tom: he had made the Blackpool finals with his previous partner, who had a good reputation, and he'd been taught by teachers all around the country. I knew that it would be an exciting step in the right direction if he said yes to dancing with me – in fact, it would be a massive jump.

Tom had tried out with other girls, but he could see how determined I was and his teacher liked me, too, which was a bonus. We instantly got on, which was important as well, because as dance partners you spend a lot of time together, dancing and travelling.

'He's way more experienced than I am,' I told Carol. 'Why would he even consider me?'

In fact, I think Tom may have been happy to partner somebody who didn't have a name, so that he could enjoy his dancing without feeling too much pressure. He was very driven and shared my aim to become a top dancer, but I got the feeling that perhaps he'd lost sight of the joy of dance and felt that he could rediscover it with me.

During the tryout, the teacher called me to one side and said, 'There's another boy available, as well. Do you know Ben Jones? I think you two would look great together.'

'I've seen him,' I said. 'I emailed him to ask for a tryout and he hasn't replied to me. So I guess it's a no.'

Weeks later, I heard from Ben. 'I'm really sorry. Your email went into my junk box. Would you still like a tryout?' I'm not quite sure I believe him, to this day! But by then I'd decided to go with Tom, partly because with Tom I'd still be eligible to enter the under-21s, which I wouldn't be with Ben, who was older, so I turned him down.

Tom and I danced well together from the start. It was a bit of a slog at first, because he lived in Walsall in the Midlands and I was still working full-time for Barratt Homes. I was driving to Birmingham and back to train with Tom one or two nights a week; he was coming to me the other nights; and then I'd drive to him on a Friday and spend the weekend having lessons and going to competitions around the country.

Actually, when I say it was *a bit* of a slog, it was completely exhausting! Eventually, I had to leave my job, partly because I kept getting ill and spending time in hospital. I moved to working part-time for Nick Lewis, a family friend, at his medical services company in Caerphilly, and started teaching Zumba classes in Birmingham. Then, as time went on and my teaching took off, I began staying with Tom and his family from Tuesday to Sunday, which made it much easier. As our partnership gelled, a relationship developed and we became girlfriend and boyfriend, which was really nice.

What made me happiest about dancing with Tom was having the opportunity to do lessons with his teachers in London, and to go to workshops and competitions I'd never had the chance to go to before. Philip and Carol have been my mentors from day one and still are, to this day, but I knew I needed to experience a range of coaching influences in order to succeed. It seemed to be working, too, and quite soon after we got together, Tom and I went to Blackpool for the Champions of Tomorrow competition and made the final in the under-21s group. My first Blackpool final! We came fifth, which seemed to confirm that we were a good pairing.

And Tom was great. My health was not good and he totally got it: he and his family were so helpful and understanding; they never made me feel guilty about missing out on competitions, even though of course he missed them too. I wasn't half as patient as they were, though. Every opportunity I had to pass up made me more anxious to go to London to see the specialist consultant that I'd been referred to.

At last the day came and I went to meet the consultant in the spring of 2009, with Mum and Dad. And that's when I learned something about doctors – they're as individual as the rest of us and some of them are really amazing people. The specialist consultant took one look at me, read a page of my notes and asked me a few questions. 'I know what's wrong with you before we even do any tests,' he said. 'You've got Crohn's disease.'

I don't think many people celebrate when they are diagnosed with a chronic illness, but it was a champagne moment for us. *Thank God!* we thought. There was just such a sense of relief that somebody had finally listened to us and believed us.

'We're going to get you on track so you can put your life back together,' he added.

He seemed so confident about it that my life completely changed from that moment, thanks to him. I wish I could name him here, because he was my saviour and I will be forever grateful to him, but he would rather stay under the radar and focus on his patients.

✦

I had to spend six whole weeks in the London hospital with the specialist consultant in the end. It was going to be two weeks, but he didn't want to let me go until he'd explored everything about my condition and tried to find the right treatment for me.

Once again I was back on a hospital ward, staring at a clock. My mum took time off work and spent the first two weeks with me, and after that she and Dad came up every weekend, but the rest of the time it was hard being on my own in an unfamiliar hospital in the middle of an unknown city. I hardly saw the outside world that May – I went for a couple of walks, but couldn't venture far with cannulas stuck in my arm, and the one time I tried to stay the night at my Auntie Carol's house in London, I had excruciating pain in my stomach and had to be rushed back to hospital.

It's tough being in a hospital bed, scrolling through Facebook and seeing all your mates at university, having the time of their lives. Not that I was bothered about going out clubbing or partying, because that has never been me, and I had chosen dancing over uni, so I accepted that I wouldn't be going into further education. I was longing to get into a dance studio, though! The worst of it was missing the British Open Championships in Blackpool, the biggest ballroom and Latin championships in the world. That made me cry, especially as Tom and I been hoping to get into the finals of the under-21s.

I followed the championships every day online. I played a game with myself to make the days more interesting: in the mornings I would wake up on the ward and imagine what

I'd be doing if I were in Blackpool: getting ready, doing my make-up, getting my hair done, putting on my dress, and trying to calm my nerves. I studied photos of the other dancers' costumes – especially Katya Jones's – and scrutinised their make-up and hair, lashes and tans. I designed new outfits in my head, inspired by Katya's, which really stood out because of the colours she put together and their diamanté patterns. She was adventurous, she didn't hold back and I loved that.

Next year I'll be there, I vowed.

Still, I knew being in hospital was the right thing for me. Even though it was tough, it meant I could get my health under control and start on the path to long-term recovery. And I was lucky: Tom stood by me and waited for me, and there's not many male dancers in our industry who would have done that.

✦

During those six weeks in London, I had an MRI scan and all the diagnostic tests I needed. When it was confirmed that I had Crohn's disease, my journey with medication started.

I thought that as soon as I was diagnosed and given medication, everything would be fine. I think I was a bit deluded in that sense: I didn't realise that it would take a few years of trial and error with different drugs to find out which were going to work for me. There aren't any short cuts: you try a certain medication for six to twelve weeks to see if it's going to work, and if it doesn't, you try something else. Everybody's experience of Crohn's is different, so the treatment has to be individually tailored to you.

My specialist consultant decided to treat my two

issues – the Crohn's disease and the severe chronic constipation – separately. First, he focused on the Crohn's, hoping that my bowel would then start to move. But it didn't, because the nerves and muscles in my large intestine had completely given up due to not having to function in the year that I'd been giving myself enemas. It would be like not using your arm for a whole year: the muscles would be completely weakened. But while you can train your arm to start lifting weight again, strengthening the muscles in the large intestine is a bit more of a challenge.

To find out more, I swallowed a pill that takes photos every two seconds until it passes right through you. In a healthy digestive system, it would take two to five days to pass through the body, but it took two whole weeks for it to pass through me – that's how sluggish my digestive system was. In the process, they discovered that my large intestine was completely paralysed. This posed a dilemma, because treating the paralysis might irritate the gut and trigger an attack of Crohn's. So what to do? The specialist consultant looked at putting in a gastric pacemaker to stimulate the bowel, but if it went on to cause inflammation of my Crohn's it could make me incontinent. I definitely didn't want to take that risk.

One day, he sat me on a bed near the toilet and tried to stimulate a bowel movement by giving me an extremely large dose of laxatives. 'We're going to do this once and if it doesn't work, we won't bother ever again,' he said. Unfortunately, I just threw them all up.

I've not opened my bowels on my own since I was nineteen, and I think the specialist consultant holds my original doctors partly responsible for giving me antidiarrhoeal agents over such a long time before I was referred for further investigations. When he heard I was given an irrigation kit and sent home without a nurse showing me how to use it, he was disgusted. I did think about suing them, but litigation is a long, gruelling process and I felt that my family and I had been through so much already. I just wanted to leave the heartache behind and get on with my life and dancing, so I chose to focus on the future, on rebuilding my life and chasing my dreams.

I made a decision and I think of it every day: don't get bitter, get better.

I learned a lot from those long years of not feeling I was being heard or believed by my doctors. One thing: my parents are saints! They taught me never to give up. Another thing: not all doctors are as caring or knowledgeable as you might think they are, but you can find the good ones, as long as you don't let yourself be fobbed off or intimidated. Ask for a second opinion. And if you don't get one, keep asking. Keep records of everything that happens in your treatment – not so you can take legal action, but so you can fight for the solution you need and deserve if it's out there. There are many wonderful staff working for the NHS. Don't stop believing in your recovery if you think you're not getting the care or information you know is available.

Some things you have to accept, unfortunately: I've had to accept that my intestine is paralysed and I've also had to accept that there isn't a cure for Crohn's disease, although a vaccine is being developed and it's looking hopeful. A lot of people with Crohn's have an operation to divert part of the bowel through an opening in the tummy, which is called a stoma, or colostomy, and involves putting a pouch over the opening to collect your poo. I feel thankful that I've been able to manage my Crohn's with medication and a strict diet so far, and avoided surgery.

There are a lot of unknowns with Crohn's and I'll always have to live with uncertainty. But, when you think about it, uncertainty is the only thing you can be certain of in life. Tomorrow is not promised to any of us. All you can do is live a life of hope, going for your goals and working hard to make them happen.

When I left the London hospital, the dreams I'd put on hold started to resurface, brighter and bolder, and Tom and I went on to have some brilliant times dancing together. I'd learned the hard way not to take things for granted. To grab your chances while you can, because they can disappear at any moment. I was determined that nothing was going to stop me. I knew what it felt like to have my dancing taken away from me, so I was going to take advantage of every minute I was well. I threw myself at every opportunity that came my way.

It took a while to sort out the right medication, but I was so much better and more hopeful when I left the London hospital that it already felt like a new lease of life. I put every last drop of energy into competing, and the fact that I'd suffered real fatigue, pain and sickness – and come out the other side – probably meant I could push a little harder in the training room, too, physically and mentally.

Tom and I got some good results in competition, but the

main thing for me was that we practised loads and had lots of lessons, and my dancing improved. The frustrated dancer inside me was finally able to learn and progress, and I was also getting my name out there a bit more. It made me so happy to feel I was making the most of the times I was healthy.

I sometimes wonder, if I hadn't had Crohn's, would I have achieved what I have? I don't know the answer, but I think it has helped define me as a person. I would never have said so in my teenage years, or even in my early twenties, but now I'm older and, looking back, I can see that it has changed me and made me stronger and more determined than I already was.

You can look at it another way, though. Dancing was my passion and gave me something to strive for. If I hadn't wanted to dance so much, and if my dream of dancing hadn't kept me going through all the tough times, would that have left me in a different place with my Crohn's? Again, I don't know.

What I do know is that the strength I developed over all those years of having Crohn's helped me get through cancer later, and so did my determination to get better and dance again.

Chapter 4

Go with your heart and the rest will follow

What's the secret of success? I never thought there was anything secret about it, if I'm honest. To me, it seemed obvious that a combination of talent, ambition, persistence, hard work, focus, energy and effort would get you there. And determination, of course. All my life I'd been telling people, 'I'm going to make it as a dancer.' I never wavered, never stopped believing.

But now I was twenty-one. I'd been dancing with Tom for two years and we weren't achieving what we wanted to achieve. We'd had some good results, but they were never amazing, and we weren't getting into any finals. Worse, we'd often go to a competition and get knocked out in the first or second round. Something was missing. I wanted more.

I could tell my parents were thinking, *She's chucked away university for this?* 'How are you going to make it now, Amy?' they asked me. 'Don't you think it's maybe too late?'

I could see why they thought time was running out. Having outgrown the under-21s, it was now time to make the jump into the adult amateur category, where the standard of dancing was miles higher. I was up against dancers who had been coached from a young age and won junior titles; they'd had a million lessons, competed in the under-12s, under-16s and under-21s and built up a name with judges and sponsors in the industry. As I didn't have those titles and that experience behind me, and nobody really knew who Tom and I were, in what universe were we suddenly going to explode onto the scene and start making it into the finals of the amateurs' group? There was no getting away from it: we were at a disadvantage.

Yet I still loved every minute of it. Yes, I'd be gutted in a competition when they missed our numbers and we didn't get through, but everything about dancing made me happy: the lessons, the practice, the dresses and dancing on the floor. It was exciting. It lit a fire in my heart. I wasn't giving up.

I think Mum and Dad were quite concerned about me at this point. They were worried I wouldn't know when to admit defeat and start adjusting my goals to a different reality. They also knew how determined I was; they knew that if I wanted something, I would put everything into making sure I got it. And I had wanted to be the best dancer in the country ever since I'd first walked into Shappelles dance school in Caerphilly, aged eight. Their fear was that I was setting myself up for sadness and disappointment in the long run. So many factors were out of my control – from my Crohn's setbacks and rising costs, to the judges' opinions on the day. They were worried that I would end up banging my head against a brick wall because I didn't know when to throw in the towel.

Then I found myself at a crossroads when my relationship with Tom broke down. Although we stayed good friends and agreed to go on dancing together after the breakup, when he met someone else and started to want different things, our dance partnership came to a natural end. That's just the way it goes, I guess – I felt we didn't share the same goals any more.

Luckily, it was an amicable split. I'm still friends with his family and I'll never forget how they stuck by me during my health problems, when they could easily have decided I wasn't worth the trouble. Not for one moment did I forget how fortunate I was to have a close-knit loving family, friends and teachers around me.

But now I was unattached again. Footloose and partner-free. 'What are you going to do now, Amy?' my parents asked.

Well, obviously I wanted to find a new partner and make my name in the amateur adult category! And then, maybe later down the line, I'd go professional, which isn't all that different from dancing in the amateur section, so I wasn't in a hurry to get there. At the same time, I recognised that I was so far from achieving my dreams that I needed a back-up plan. 'If, by the age of twenty-five, I haven't made it as a dancer,' I promised myself, 'I'll go to university and become a primary school teacher.'

There. I'd done it. I had somewhere to go if things went wrong – and a few more years to prove myself.

Then along came Ben Jones.

✦

Ben and I had barely spoken since he'd emailed me for a tryout, two years earlier. We'd say, 'Good luck', or, 'How are you today?', but nothing more. We'd competed against each other – we were rivals – and one or two coaches had suggested that we'd make a good pair, so we were still conscious of each other in that way, too. After I'd split with Tom, I was watching

Ben dancing at a competition one weekend and started thinking they might be right. I knew his mum a little bit as she's a very bubbly people's person and used to go round chatting to everyone at competitions, so I went over to have a chat with her. 'I'd love to try out with Ben if the chance ever comes up,' I told her.

Although he already had a partner, I had the feeling he might like to have a go at dancing with me. The next thing I knew, we were in the studio having a tryout. It was exciting because he's a very talented dancer (and looks good, too!). But I tried to keep a lid on my hopes. I had to accept that the boys have all the power in our industry. Anything could happen.

And something did happen: Ben was fun to dance with. He had me giggling straight away and we could instantly tell that we'd work well together. We were a good match physically, too: Ben is a very masculine dancer and I'm quite feminine, and I need somebody powerful.

Ben had started dancing later than most, at fifteen, when he took his sister to her dance lessons and the teachers persuaded him to have a go. I think he only agreed because he fancied one of the girls in the class! Then it only took a few weeks for the teachers to spot how much promise he had and he progressed very quickly.

Being a late starter meant that, like me, although for different reasons, he didn't have any junior titles or connections in the dance industry. Neither of us were 'pedigree', so if we became a couple, I knew we'd have to work extra hard, especially as Ben wasn't interested in cosying up to judges or coaches. He made it clear from the start that he wanted to get to the top because of his own talent and merit. Being a hard worker myself, I liked that about him.

We danced every day for a week, which is standard for a tryout, and by the end of it, I knew I wanted to dance with Ben. But he wasn't letting on. And I couldn't push it, as he was already in a couple.

I was in the Peacocks store in Caerphilly with my best friend, Kate, when he rang me and said, 'I'd like to dance with you, Amy.'

'Amazing!' I burst out. It was the best news. I started texting all my friends and family to say, 'Yeah, I'm going to dance with Ben!'

I was still in the middle of texting people when he rang me back. 'Er, I've changed my mind,' he told me. 'I can't split with my partner. I can't do it to her.'

My heart plummeted. 'Wha—?' I couldn't believe what I was hearing. Then I remembered I'd told his mum about my Crohn's disease and immediately thought that must be the reason he'd changed his mind.

He burst out laughing. 'Only joking!'

Oh no, I thought, trying to catch my breath. *What have I let myself in for?*

'Actually, I was just ringing to see if you're coming to practice tonight,' he said.

I relaxed. 'Yeah, if you want me to, I can come up, no problem.'

At the practice, we talked about the British National Dance Championships in Blackpool, in six weeks' time.

'Pity it's too soon for us,' I said, regretfully.

Our eyes met. His gaze was piercing and I knew what he was thinking. *Let's give it a shot. Why not?*

Normally, you'd wait a couple of months before you started

competing; you'd bond as a partnership, connect and get your routines sorted. But we decided to go for it.

'We'll need to practise every day . . .' I said, transfixed by his blue eyes.

He grinned. 'Great!'

✦

Ben's parents, Simon and Elaine, were building a bungalow in the garden of their house in Dudley in the West Midlands. It was for his nan to live in, and Ben asked them if I could share it with her. They were surprised, because he had never wanted a dance partner to move in with him before. Any non-dancers reading this might be wondering why he didn't come and live with me. Well, he would have been welcome – but that never happens in the dance industry! Annoyingly, the girls always go to the boys. I've never heard of it happening the other way round, even if it's overseas: I remember turning down a potential partner once because he lived in Italy and I wanted to stay in the UK. Although, in this instance, Ben's home was better positioned than mine for going to London and other parts of the country, maybe it's time for the industry to wake up to the fact that it's the twenty-first century now?

I stayed in Ben's family's house while the bungalow was being built. Sadly, his nan passed away before it was finished, so his other nan, Pauline, moved into it instead and I went on to share it with her. Pauline is lovely; she did my washing for me sometimes and we used to enjoy having a cup of tea and a chat at the end of the day. And I do love my cups of tea.

Staying with Ben meant that I got to know him on fast-forward: instead of meeting up to dance and then going our separate ways, we were living in each other's pockets. I guess it was only a matter of a time before we began to fall in love.

His parents were the first to think something was going on between us. They started hearing my footsteps at night as I crept into the house from the bungalow . . . We still didn't tell anyone, but my mum noticed. 'You're very giggly when you talk about Ben,' she said.

Our relationship secretly blossomed over those six weeks of intense preparation for the Blackpool championships. We travelled to London a few times a week for lessons with three different coaches and we sometimes went up to Liverpool for lessons with a well-known teacher, who taught a lot of top dancers. We practised in every spare moment. We knew we couldn't expect to achieve much after six weeks, but maybe we could make it to the semi-final? That was our hope. And we went all out, trying to make it happen.

We'd both had more success in the Latin American section: Ben's build is more suited to being a Latin than a ballroom dancer and I guess our personalities along with our body shapes are just more Latin. Ballroom is more a bit more refined and classy; Latin is fun and lively. As we only had six weeks to prepare, it seemed natural to focus on the Latin dances.

When the time came, the atmosphere in the Blackpool Winter Gardens was electric. My parents and Rebecca came to watch, and Ben's parents were there as well; I wore a black dress with black feathers, covered in shimmering multi-coloured crystal diamantés. I think we both felt amazing as we went out there onto the famous dance floor. It was our first competition together, everything felt right, and as we danced the rumba, I remember thinking, *Yeah, this is it.*

We gave it our best shot, and the judges must have liked us because we actually made the semi-final. Our London coach was over the moon. 'That's an unbelievable achievement for a partnership of six weeks!' he kept saying. We did really well, too: we came ninth out of hundreds of couples. It was the best result either of us had ever achieved! We were so happy and excited, because it was such a tough competition.

This is going to work, I thought, as we left the Winter Gardens afterwards. *I can become a champion. I've got the right partner. All the ingredients are there. We can do this.*

I think both sets of our parents could see it as well. You just kind of know in dancing when a couple have something special. It felt like everything had fallen into place.

A lot of it was down to Ben. All the top dancers across the world have something that sets them apart, and Ben had his own unique style and ways. He was very different from other male dancers in that he never wanted to play the political card and kiss up to the judges. His attitude was: you either like me as a dancer or you don't.

I admired that – he had his own personality and knew his own worth; he didn't just want to follow the crowd and conform. He was never thinking: *Is this what the judges want?* It was: *How am I going to express myself?* He's a proper showman on the floor, very creative. However, sometimes I was uncomfortable with it, because I'm very much a people-pleaser. So, while he was taking risks, I was worrying about the judges. He wasn't bothered, though. People in the ballroom would be walking around in suits – and I always made sure I dressed smartly and said polite hellos to everyone I passed – but he'd be wearing the clothes he wanted to wear. He was always Ben Jones. And I loved that about him.

Ben pushed me to be different. And although that took me out of my comfort zone, it brought out the best in me. Ultimately, you don't want to be like everyone else. You want to be memorable. You want to be iconic.

In dancing, you can't help but compare your dance moves and dance outfits with other people's. But just because somebody won on that day, or that dress worked in that venue, it doesn't necessarily mean it's going to work at the next competition. Why change your plan and what you believe in? Better to stay focused on what you're working towards. Believe in what your coaches are telling you and in your partnership.

You can easily get sidetracked by watching another couple. But they could have taken months and months of working on a certain thing to get to that level. Ben and I would always set ourselves goals: 'Let's work on our technique for a few weeks. Then let's work on our competition performance.'

Everyone has dips and highs. Some people show a sudden improvement, then they may plateau for a while before improving again. Meanwhile, you're just slowly getting better, step by step. So don't get distracted; keep believing in your route, your goal, your partnership and the team around you.

✦

We went on having lessons in London and Liverpool and I think one of the London coaches could see the potential in us. He was thinking, *I've got a British couple here who could go all the way.*

So he gave us a word of advice: 'Whatever you do, don't get together, because it will affect your dancing if the relationship breaks down and one of you moves on with someone else.' All the hard work – ours and the coach's – would be for nothing if we split. It happens a lot. You see couples who are about to win, who are about to become one of the most successful pairs the world has ever seen – and then their relationship breaks down and they fall apart.

He didn't want anything to get in the way. He just wanted us to be focused.

'OK,' we said.

Whoops! Too late. By then we were madly in love and there was no going back.

We tried to keep our relationship secret for years. We thought nobody knew, but *everybody* knew. They could just tell it because of how we were around each other, the way we spoke to each other and because we never left each other's side. Nobody ever bothered asking us, though – they just assumed. I think in this day and age people don't go asking, 'Are you girlfriend and boyfriend?' especially in the dancing world, because most people are couples. And if they're not, they're best friends and soulmates, so it wouldn't be surprising to see them hug or hold hands.

I spoke to Ben about my Crohn's disease when we first got together in November 2011, but as I didn't have a flare-up until three months later, about six weeks after we'd made the semi-finals at Blackpool, he probably thought it wasn't something to worry about too much. I started feeling more optimistic, too. When you have a chronic illness, you live in hope of going into remission and being symptom-free.

I've not been poorly for a little while, I thought. *Maybe it's getting better.*

Crohn's is brought on by stress and I was feeling happy and in a good place, so I'm sure that helped: I was loving what I was doing; I was in a new partnership and having an exciting time with Ben; I was trialling new medications that seemed to be managing things.

I didn't want Ben to see me have a flare-up. I was in love with him and wanted him to see me at my best. So I tried to ignore it when my energy started to dip. *No*, I thought, *I'm going to be fine. I'm so much better now.*

It was February and we were training hard for the British Open Championships in Blackpool in the spring. We were at a practice session with other couples in a church hall in Rowley Regis when suddenly I was hit by pain and collapsed. An ambulance had to be called – Ben came with me to the hospital and so did his mum. His family were a great support to me, but they were quite taken aback by how much I suffered, as was Ben.

During a Crohn's flare-up, excruciating, knife-stabbing pain takes over your entire body and you don't get a break from it. No other pain comes close. I dislocated my kneecap once and had to travel to hospital with my kneecap halfway down my leg before it was put back again – and I was fine. When my appendix burst, I thought it was a stomach bug and didn't even want to go to the doctor's. But the pain of a Crohn's flare-up is something else. You take 5ml of morphine for a broken leg or foot and it takes the pain away, but I need 20ml of morphine – four times that amount – in order to start easing the pain of

Crohn's. A woman's body is designed to cope with the pain of childbirth and it's extremely rare to faint during labour, but the pain of Crohn's is so bad that it makes me pass out, and the rest of the time I'm being sick and sweating.

When you go on the gastro ward and you hear that cry, you just know the pain they're going through, when you can't even walk, you can't even crawl to the bathroom to be sick or have diarrhoea. Often, when I start being sick, I don't leave the bathroom; I just stay on the bathroom floor because it's easier. Afterwards, I sleep for days because I am so exhausted. I hardly wake at all.

'It's unbelievable that you go through all this and still have the desire and determination to continue dancing and be the best you can!' Ben said.

Although I'd spoken about it, I guess it's completely different when you see it happen. Years later, Katya Jones, my friend and fellow dancer on *Strictly*, said that it was really eye-opening for her the first time she saw me collapse with Crohn's.

It must be tough to see someone you love in so much pain and Ben was terrified it would happen again. He was always telling me off for rushing back to training too soon after a flare-up. 'Please don't overdo it,' he would say.

'I'm fine!' I'd reassure him, even when I wasn't. 'Let's get back to training.'

I knew I was supposed to take extra care of myself and allow myself to recover gently after a flare-up, but as soon as I felt able, I'd be up and off again. I was desperate to live my life to the full when I should probably have paced myself a bit more. I'm a lot better about taking care of myself these days, but it's something I'm still learning.

✦

For the next few years, Ben and I lived together, practised and competed together and worked together teaching dance lessons and Zumba lessons. That's how it is for any couple in our dancing world, whether they're in a relationship or not. For me, I think it's helpful to be in a relationship with your dance partner. You have no outside distractions – you literally train as much as you possibly can – and you get to share your passion for dance with the person you love. Of course, you're taking a risk, but it didn't feel like there was any danger of me and Ben falling out. They say you know when you know. Well, we knew.

Ben and I complemented each other. I was the worrier and he was Mr Calm-and-Confident. He was good about moving on and forgetting a bad result, but I hated the feeling, got really upset and thought about it for weeks afterwards. Although I needed that feeling, too, because it's what gave me the fire in my belly to push hard and beat them next time, his mindset helped me get through without taking it too much to heart.

One year, we had a really bad result at a competition at the Grosvenor House hotel in the centre of London, two weeks before an important championship in Blackpool. We felt we'd danced well but it was our worst result in years and I was in tears.

'Just focus on the fact that we danced well,' Ben kept saying afterwards, but I couldn't stop going over why we hadn't got a good result. I'd worn my new black dress, which was covered in black diamantés, and a big red rose in my hair and red shoes, and everybody had complimented it, so it wasn't the dress.

'What was it?' I asked him. 'What can we change in the next two weeks before the championships?'

'Nothing,' Ben said. 'It's just the judges' opinion. At the next competition there'll be a different panel of judges and the result could be completely different. Let's be true to ourselves as dancers and be the dancers we want to be, rather than trying to second-guess what the judges like. Let's be the dancers we will always look back and be proud of.'

I was distraught all the way home while he was able to brush it off. He doesn't lose sleep over anything; he's very chilled. 'Right, we'll just get back into the studio tomorrow and work hard,' he said. 'We're not going to change our routines or anything else before Blackpool. We're just going to focus and go on believing in what we're doing.'

We went to Blackpool and beat the people who had beaten us at the Grosvenor House hotel. We went quite a few rounds further than them, in fact. So Ben was right, as usual. Frustratingly so, because he always wins in an argument.

The thing is, all dancers have good days and bad days, and maybe the other couple had been having a really good day when they danced at the Grosvenor House hotel. That's just how it goes. And sometimes, when it feels good, it doesn't always look good.

With my students, I'll say, 'That's the best you've ever done.'

'But it felt terrible!'

'Well, it looked the best.'

I wish I could say that I've learned how to shut off my anxiety, but I'm still learning. I try listening to music and other things that will distract me. There are so many lessons we learn in life, and there're so many areas we can always improve upon as a person, and my anxiety is one I still need to work on. I'm not ashamed to admit that.

What kept me going was the passion and excitement of competing, and I'd say that was another key to our success. If what you're doing gives you a buzz and a thrill (even if it's only for some of the time), you're going to be eager to put your energy and effort into it, aren't you?

There was maybe something else that was there for me and Ben, which helped us succeed. At least, I don't think we would have made it to where we are now without it. It's quite difficult to pin down. You could say that it was something in Ben's blue eyes, and that was part of it, for sure. His unique style and the way he made me giggle had a lot to do with it. The fact that he was more talented than me? I admit it: he stretched and improved my dancing. Our shared passion for dance – ups, downs and all – was also a massive part of the magic.

The fact that Ben always, without fail, put my health first when a Crohn's flare-up forced me to pull out of practising, or a competition, meant the world to me. No question about it – I was the priority and his unwavering devotion gave me the confidence to bounce back and keep going every time I was ill.

So if I had to sum it all up – and I'm not saying it has to be this way for everybody – for us, for Ben and me, I think the key ingredient to our success was love. Wholehearted, unquestioning, unlimited, out and out love and affection.

Chapter 5

Today's failure is tomorrow's lesson

Anyone chasing a dream knows that you have to make sacrifices. And it's especially true if you're going to compete at the highest level in the world of ballroom and Latin American dancing. You don't have a social life – you don't have the money or the time for one. You're squeezing in every practice you can at ridiculous hours of the day, teaching dance classes and Zumba to pay your expenses, or driving up and down the country to lessons and competitions. If I ever had a little break, which wouldn't be often, maybe once every couple of months, I'd quickly go home to Wales and see my family.

At times, it can feel like you're giving up everything. For years, Ben and I didn't have the money to go on holidays or enjoy nights out. On a weekend off, you'd often find us counting the pennies and weighing up whether we could justify the expense of going to the cinema. We were always saving for our next competition, dance lesson, costume or pair of shoes, so our treat on a Saturday night would more likely mean chilling in his bedroom and watching a film; and maybe Ben's dad would get us an Indian takeaway. I'm not complaining – I loved our treat nights, even if we were just staying in – but occasionally it would have been nice to do something different.

Most of the time we felt it was worth cutting back, so that we could spend what we had on our dancing. The cost of competing really mounts up: some of the foreign competitions can cost as much as a hundred euros per person to enter, and the big English competitions are forty or fifty pounds. And that's just the start of it: you have the fuel costs of driving at least two hours there and back; you're not working or teaching that day, so you lose income; then it's the cost of your tan, your eyelashes, your dress and hair. It's an expensive day – and if it's an international competition, add on your flights and hotel.

We didn't get sponsored until towards the end of our competing career, so at Christmas and birthdays I always said the same thing to my parents: 'Can I have some money towards a new pair of dance shoes?' Or Mum might give me some fake eyelashes or fake tan – any of the things you need to compete.

Ben's parents helped a lot, too, and thanks to them, we didn't have to pay household bills or rent, as we still lived at their house. They wanted us to do well and fitted their family life and calendar around our competitions; they washed our dance costumes for us and put up with us coming in late and getting our meals ready every night after training. They helped us in so many ways. They even bought me a new car after I ran my old car into the ground in the first year because it was so much cheaper on fuel than Ben's was.

I'm not sure how long we could have kept going if our family and friends hadn't been so understanding. My sister was an amazing support, especially after she left university and started working as a midwife. While I was still only just getting by, she would buy my next dance dress and I'd pay her back in monthly instalments. Everyone helped out.

✦

Going without material things was never easy, but my biggest problem was feeling homesick. On a basic level, I missed living in Wales. I love England and the rest of the UK, but I feel very Welsh and am proud of it, too. I love the Welsh culture of music and poetry. I love the countryside – the mountains, the sea and the sense of space. I was homesick for it all.

And I missed my home town of Caerphilly, where everybody knows everybody and I can't go anywhere without bumping into somebody I know. The Welsh stick together and it's like one massive family in Caerphilly. The feeling that I belong is very strong; I'll go into the bank and someone will say, 'Oh look, it's one of the twins!' and it's always nice to stop and chat. However long I've been away, when I'm back it doesn't feel like more than two minutes since I was last there.

Most of all, I missed my family: my mum and dad, who are still so in love after all these years and who do everything together; my brother, Lloyd, who spent his childhood putting up with my noise and sparkly dresses; and my best friend and twin sister, Rebecca. Not to mention our wider family and friends, who always welcome me back with open arms, no matter how long it's been since I've seen them.

When I was growing up, it didn't bother me too much to miss out on birthday parties, sleepovers and hanging out with friends, because I would always rather be dancing; but I felt it more as I got older and had to forfeit weekends away with the family for dance training and practice. I've missed a lot of family birthdays over the years, which is hard for someone as family focused as me; I even had to skip my dad's sixtieth a few years ago. That was hard. My dad is such a fun guy, the one everyone wants on their table; he's a joker, always up to mischief, and he loves good times. So although I was enjoying rehearsals for *Strictly* at the time, I was gutted not to be with him, having fun. I couldn't go to my best friend Kate's wedding in Dubai, either, because it fell on the same weekend as the British Open Championships in Blackpool (and, also, I couldn't have afforded to get there). But missing out is something I've just had to accept; it goes with the territory. You have to be prepared to give things up.

There were times in my early twenties when I felt ground down by it all. I missed my family and friends in Caerphilly; Ben and I were constantly scrimping and worrying about money. Every day was a race to earn enough cash to keep going.

But I knew it would be worth it in the end, if I could just keep going.

Anyway, making sacrifices drives you to work harder and appreciate what you have. I wasn't someone who took things for granted, and going without always made me think, *One day, I'll be able to afford the nice things in life. Don't give up . . .*

I kept my optimism by staying focused on my long-term dreams. Yes, there will be bumps along the road, but it's important to remember that now isn't your ultimate goal, so if you do badly at something, it doesn't matter, because there's always tomorrow. Every champion has been through heartache.

I knew that if I didn't make the necessary sacrifices, I might regret it – and no one wants to live with regret and look back and think, *I wish I'd done that*. Because you can't change the past.

So we just had to grit our teeth and get on with it. And whenever we gave ourselves a treat, we made sure we savoured it – even if it was just a bottle of wine and some posh crisps at the weekend.

Through it all, I tried to see the bigger picture and keep hold of my dreams, imagining what it would feel like if I achieved them. It helped that Ben and I were a team. We were sacrificing everything, but we were doing it together. It probably wouldn't have worked if one did and the other didn't, because we needed each other's support. I don't know how people do it without a partner by their side; athletes in individual sports have a much harder time of it.

In our first year together, we really slogged hard: working all hours to pay for lessons in London and practising whenever we could. It often felt as if we weren't getting anywhere, though, just hovering around the quarters and semis in competitions. Sometimes I just wanted to cry out to the judges, 'I've given up my whole life for this! Can't you see?'

After a bad result, I'd go very quiet and maybe ring Mum and Dad and let out my disappointment on the journey home. Ben would quickly bounce back, but sometimes I'd feel sad and angry and *just so frustrated*, and there would be a low mood in the Jones household that evening. Mostly, though, we'd put on some good music on the way home in the car, have a good chat and focus on what we needed to do better. We learned a lot from the bad results. They taught us far more than the good results did – and probably gave us the kick that we needed.

Once we were home, we'd study videos from the competition in order to see what we needed to do better, and the following morning, we'd be eager to be back in the studio practising. That's the good thing about dancing – there are so many competitions in your diary that you've always got something new to focus on. Look to the future. Don't dwell on the past: you can't change it; you can't do anything about it.

Sheer hard work went into trying for a good result. Right, I'm going to show you, I'd think.

I constantly kept in mind that motto on the banner in our assembly hall at school, 'Fail to prepare, prepare to fail.' I knew that if we didn't work on our fitness and our stamina, we weren't going to be able to go out there and dance five dances back to back at the level we wanted to. Now, there's no point in having all those lessons on technique – all those lessons learning to spin super fast and do other tricks – when you haven't worked on your stamina to be able to execute it. This is something I say to all my students, and I apply my school motto to everything I do. I wouldn't go into *Strictly* without having prepared my choreography, or into a meeting about music choices with my celebrity partner without some ideas about the theme of our routine. Having that banner above me every day in assembly and reading it every morning just kind of stuck with me.

When people watch you on a competition floor doing a beautiful dance routine, they don't see the months and months of hard work it took to get there. The work it takes to get your body looking a certain way, as good as the muscular

Eastern European girls; your work on your fitness levels; or even the effort that goes into picking your dresses, hairstyles and make-up. And that's the way it's supposed to be. When you're dancing at the highest level, the audience and the judges will only see the lovely dances you've just done, not the blood, sweat and tears that went into perfecting them.

✦

Dancers often specialise around the age of twenty-one because no one can make it at the top levels of both Latin American and ballroom. If you try, you'll only end up as jack of all trades and master of none. While there is a ten-dance section, far fewer couples compete in it, and no one from the ten-dance section has made it yet to the finals of the ballroom or Latin American championships. They'd be more likely to make it to the last forty-eight or twenty-four. When you're going up against somebody who specialises in putting all of their time, effort and coaching into either Latin or ballroom, while you're splitting your time between all ten dances, with the best will in the world you're not going to match their level.

After doing so well in our first Blackpool Nationals together, and being at that age where we would need to specialise anyway, and also not having loads of money to pay for double the lessons – for both ballroom and Latin – Ben and I made a decision. Or Ben did, anyway. 'I know I said I would do ballroom as well, but I want to focus on Latin,' he said, and I'm glad he made the decision for us because I don't think I would have ever been able to choose, as I loved them both equally.

A year after we surprised ourselves by coming ninth in the British National Dance Championships, we went back to

Blackpool hoping to make the final in the Latin American section. After working so, so hard and giving up so, so much, surely this would be our breakthrough?

It wasn't. We ended up with a worse result than the year before and went home heartbroken. It felt as if we hadn't made any progress in a whole year of dancing together. We still had such a long way to go.

I was so devastated that I asked my mum to come up to Birmingham and spend the day with me. I felt really low, really homesick, and Mum remembers it as being the one time she thought I was ready to pack it all in. Ben was the same: we'd spent all that money on coaching and given up everything in our lives, and we couldn't see how we were ever going to rise up to be champions.

'What are you going to do next?' Mum asked gently. 'Why don't you ask Neil and Katya for some advice?'

Neil and Katya Jones were the couple we adored and looked up to on the competition circuit. And not only did we love their style, but they were also winning a lot of titles. They're now on *Strictly*, of course, but at the time they were working with a coach called Richard Porter, so we thought we'd reach out to him and see if he would teach us, too.

Richard is an international Latin dance champion and trained choreographer who's been in demand as a coach ever since he retired from professional dancing in his late twenties. He had just judged the competition at Blackpool, so it seemed a good moment. We messaged him saying, 'Hey, we'd love to book a lesson with you. You judged us last week at the British National Championships. We were in blue and we made the semi-final.'

'Hi, don't remember you, at all,' was his reply.

That was hard (especially the devastating position of that second comma!). This was a coach who only ever worked with champions. Still, he said he would take a look at us. And he would be able to decide after that lesson if he was interested, as would we.

The following weekend, he said, 'I have a cancellation next Saturday in London.'

We went down to London knowing that this was going to be the decider for both of us. Everything depended on our lesson with Richard: if he agreed to coach us, we would continue dancing; if not, we probably wouldn't, and I'd apply for teacher training.

I was super nervous. Would he laugh us out of the studio? All kinds of possibilities went through my head: he would halt the lesson after five minutes; he would shake his head and say, 'I'm sorry. There's nothing I can do for you.' He would look at us bleakly and tell us he'd be in touch soon, never to call . . .

Don't be silly, I told myself. I banished every negative scenario from my head and gave myself a pep talk. Just go and see if you like his style of teaching, first – if we get on and if it's meant to be. Relax. Breathe. You have forty-five minutes in which to impress him. You can do this.

The lesson turned out to be amazing and we loved it. Right from the start, we were both thinking the same: *We need this coach. If we don't work with him, we're not going to make it.*

When the session ended, I was desperate to know what Richard was thinking, too. There was a long pause before he finally spoke.

It happened that he had an opening for a new couple, he

said, because Neil and Katya had just retired from amateur dancing to become professionals.

Yes, and . . . ?

'And I actually think we could work together,' he concluded.

'Really?' A jolt of excitement went through me.

'Let's make sure the title passes from one Jones to another Jones,' Ben and I joked, in relief.

Richard smiled. 'The only problem is that I'm moving to America, next month.' Oh, no. My heart dropped down to my Cuban heels. He continued, 'So you'd have to come to LA for your lessons.'

Ben and I exchanged worried glances. We'd be unlikely to afford regular flights to America, but maybe, *maybe* we might be able to borrow money from someone to help towards the cost. It would mean tightening our belts even more than ever, though.

'I'll let you think about it, but I'll give you a slot in my diary if you want it.'

Wow, that in itself was a huge thing.

Would it be worth all that effort and outlay, though? The sacrifices we'd have to make? We asked Richard for an honest opinion of our chances. 'We want to win,' we told him.

He looked serious. 'I think you could make it,' he said. 'I really think you could do it.'

✦

Back home in Birmingham, we weren't sure where to turn. Ben's parents, Simon and Elaine, had already gone above and beyond for us. Simon had his own company and worked very, very hard. How could we load even more pressure on him by asking him for money? I knew my parents would have contributed if they were able, but it just wasn't possible. Who could we ask, not knowing when we could pay them back or if we'd ever achieve our dream of winning the Nationals in Blackpool?

It was Ben's dad, Simon, who saved the day. He could see in Ben's eyes how much Ben wanted to work with Richard. He knew that we thought working with Richard was our only way to get to the top. 'I'll help you. I'll pay for your flights,' he offered. 'Just say yes, and we'll sort it out from here.' Without Simon's generosity, who knows what would have happened. It was an incredible act of kindness that I won't forget.

Things became exciting after that. We worked the hardest we've ever worked to pay for lessons and accommodation in LA, where we went to see Richard Porter every other month. Being in LA was time to rest and recuperate from our frantic schedule back in England, where I was teaching five different Zumba classes and teaching dance in local schools. Ben and I were doing everything we could from month to month to get to those lessons with Richard. At times it impacted my health, as it was incredibly stressful trying to earn enough money to cover the cost of each trip. A lesson with Richard cost $250 for forty-five minutes, and we had a minimum of ten lessons every time we went to LA, so it was a huge outlay.

It was worth it, though, because training with Richard transformed our dancing. Here was a coach who fully believed in us, and also cared about us. Richard took us on as nobodies and helped us make a name for ourselves. He truly wanted us to do well and completely changed our routine.

He could be savage sometimes; he was brutally honest with

us and often had me in tears, stopping the music and saying, 'Again, again, again.' He'd take me to breaking point – and Ben had it just as bad – because he knew that ultimately this was how to make me the best dancer. Sometimes we would leave his lesson crying, but we still loved him – it was weird.

My sister used to be outraged on my behalf. 'The way he's just spoken to you, the messages he's sent – I don't know why you're spending that much money with him! It's ridiculous.'

But we knew he was the best teacher for us. He didn't just teach us and take our money, like other coaches we knew – which was fair enough, they did what we paid them to do – Richard cared about every single one of our competitions and performances, right down to our costumes and routines. All his other couples already had a name for themselves. I think he wanted to take a couple of diamonds in the rough and make them into something. We were the raw stones that Richard cut and polished, and it was painful sometimes.

After one competition, I remember asking him, 'How do you think I did?'

'You didn't turn up,' he said curtly.

'I did, I was in the black dress with the bows!'

'You didn't turn up and dance, though, did you? Ben, how does it feel that your partner didn't actually show up?'

Richard may have been sharp and unforgiving in class, but we got the sense that he was looking out for us even outside our lessons. We began to forge a special connection; every time we went to LA, knowing that we couldn't afford to go out, Richard would take us somewhere lovely. Once, when we were competing in Holland, I saw a dress I wanted to wear the following week in Blackpool. It was bright orange, with stones and beads on one side and plain fabric on the other. It was unique and expensive, and Richard gave me the money to buy it, knowing I couldn't stretch to buying it myself. 'Pay it back when you can. Don't worry about it,' he said.

We stopped going to our teachers in London. We couldn't afford to do both and we'd totally given ourselves over to Richard. A lot of the professionals didn't like that. Some people took offence that a British couple were going to another country for lessons. They saw it as meaning that we thought they weren't good enough teachers, but it wasn't that. We'd been going to lessons in London for a year and just needed a completely fresh approach. It was all or nothing with Richard, basically.

At first, it was nothing. Richard helped us towards a whole new dancing mentality, but it took time, and we saw a massive dip in our results at the start. We had to get worse to get better, we told ourselves, and tried not to feel discouraged. If Richard Porter thought we had something special, we just had to keep believing.

Even though we went on to have a terrible result at the UK championships in Bournemouth in the summer of 2013, we kept pushing ourselves. The judges weren't keen on us that day – so on to the next! Then, in the October, we went to a competition in the Midlands where lots of top international couples go to compete before the international championships at the Royal Albert Hall. I think our previous placing must have freed our minds somehow and when we went out onto the dance floor at this competition, we weren't really thinking about our result. We were there to enjoy ourselves.

Then a really extraordinary thing happened. To our absolute surprise, the announcer called us into first place. First place? We weren't at all prepared when they announced it. And, even then, we couldn't compute. 'Wha—? We've won? You're joking!'

How did that happen? We hadn't even made the final at the UK championships in Bournemouth, and now we'd beaten every couple who'd taken part in that final, bar one. It left us reeling with shock and confusion amid the elation. The other British couples weren't placed just behind us, either. We came first, then there were several international couples, and below them were the other British couples. It was the weirdest thing. We just couldn't work it out. It gave us the boost we needed, at just the right time, and a massive sense of relief, because our results until then had been so awful. I felt like a kid at Christmas and it was the best feeling in the world. Finally, we'd made our breakthrough.

Everything felt different after that. All of a sudden, it seemed, our names were on the map. Judges, competitors and professionals all saw us as contenders. Our results dramatically changed. At the British National Dance Championships at Blackpool the year before, we'd just about scraped into the semi-final; the following year, we were announced into the final. It was a massive jump. We made it into the final the following year, too, and started getting international results. Everything began to take off for us.

My first sponsorship deal came in 2015 when Brad, a wonderfully creative designer at the dancewear company Studio Armell, designed a dress for me. Brad had worked under a designer whose dresses I often wore and I met him in Blackpool just as he was starting his own business.

'Would you do a photo shoot for me, Amy?' he asked. 'I'd love it if you became part of my team.'

I was thrilled. And maybe because he was one of the first to believe in us and give us sponsorship, a beautiful friendship began to develop and now he's one of our best friends. He still designs all my show and competition dance dresses to this day, and the kids' costumes at our dance studio as well.

In November 2015, Ben and I went to Blackpool again for the British National Dance Championships – 'the Nationals' – hoping to make the final, even though it didn't look like a particularly good panel of judges for us, as most of them hadn't rated us highly in past competitions.

In dancing, your results depend on experts' opinions. There's no science to it, no right or wrong – you don't cross the line first, or jump the highest. It's purely based on the experts' individual viewpoints and whether or not they like what you're doing. And obviously that can go for or against you.

Back then, it was well known that if a couple did a lot of political manoeuvring, they'd have an advantage. I'm talking about the sort of couple who went from judge to judge for lessons, making a name for themselves, and whose parents were pally with the judges and sat with them during the competitions. As Ben and I weren't ever going to go down the political route and become industry darlings, even if we could have, coming up against couples like this was very frustrating – although I'm glad to say that the dance world is a lot fairer in this respect now.

We couldn't have been happier when we were announced into the final that year. But although we'd been getting great results in recent months, we weren't expecting to get beyond fifth or sixth place. (The best possible result would be second place, as ballroom tradition dictates that last year's winners always come first, until they retire from the category.)

I was twenty-five now and conscious of the back-up plan I'd made four years earlier. It wasn't that we'd given up on becoming champions, but I was beginning to think that maybe we didn't have the money, pedigree or connections to go all the way to the top. However, nothing and no one could take away our passion for dancing.

Who cares? we were thinking, as we went out and danced that night. *Let's just be true to ourselves, and if they don't like it, then let's at least dance for us, and for the love of dancing.*

We had such low expectations that it was like dynamite exploding when they called out our names for second place. We were totally blown away, because second place is as good as first place in the dancing world. It means you're on a trajectory to winning. Out of the blue, we had made it.

'Ben, we did it!' I screamed, jumping up and down like a maniac and making noises that were only half-human.

As we ran onto the floor, Ben broke down in tears – tears of joy, relief and years of pent-up frustration. We had worked so hard, for so long, and now, at last, the judges had realised how much our dancing meant to us. We just wanted to dance.

The entire ballroom could see how much that result meant to Ben and me. The champion, Petar Daskalov, from

Denmark, went up to Ben and shook his hand. 'Ben, I should be crying, not you,' he said wryly.

In the dance newspaper that goes out worldwide once a week, the front page photo of the line-up showed all the winners smiling and Ben just crying his eyes out. It quickly became a meme and our shoe sponsors, International Dance Shoes, who had only recently given us a sponsorship deal, sent Ben a box of Kleenex tissues and a pair of shoes with the letters CB stitched on, short for 'Cry Baby'. It really made us laugh.

For us, that UK championship result in 2015 was the highpoint of our whole dancing career, even though we came second. It was so unexpected for us, and for our family and our friends. We'd taken another massive jump and it was exhilarating to think that the risks we'd taken, the sacrifices we'd made and all those hours and hours of practice had paid off. We couldn't wait to take a shot at the title the following year.

'Next stop, the World Championships!' our coach Richard said, with a smile. 'Don't forget you're going to Paris next week.'

'Oh no, we can't afford it,' I said.

Before our surprise result at the Nationals, we hadn't been planning to go to the World Championships, mainly because of the expense, yet now we didn't really have a choice, because the top two British couples at the British National Dance Championships are automatically selected to go to the World Championships. But where would we find the funds for our travel and hotel? We were already overdrawn and down to our last few pounds of borrowed money.

Once again, Ben's parents kindly helped us out. Competing in Paris was their Christmas present to us, and we were so thankful.

We practised all day every day in the run-up, but had a setback two days before the competition started: I broke my thumb and it was very, very painful. But nothing could stop me from dancing, so I bandaged it up and we changed the hand connections in the routine to put less strain on it.

To our amazement we were announced into the quarter-finals of the World Championships. It was another big jump for us and we were buzzing. It was astonishing to go so much further than we expected, two weeks in a row!

Richard Porter popped down to see us. 'Amy, can you dance without the bandage on your thumb? It's distracting, and you guys are on fire tonight.'

Ben shook his head. 'We don't want the break to get any worse,' he said, bless him.

'Come on, let's do it,' I coaxed. 'It's for only one round.'

One round wouldn't make a difference, I figured, and we knew we weren't going to make it further than the quarter-finals. The top twenty-four couples in the world were competing, and we weren't *ever* going to beat them. It was amazing enough to be sharing a space with them.

So we took to the floor and danced the quarter-finals, and as the adrenalin kicked in, I couldn't feel the pain of my broken thumb at all.

'I loved that!' I said afterwards, hugging Ben.

He couldn't stop grinning. 'Amazing, wasn't it?'

Richard came up to speak to us again. 'I think you should warm up, guys, for the semi-final,' he said.

We looked at him in surprise. 'What? We've never even made the quarter-finals before. There's no way we are ever going to make it to the semis of the World Championships.' I looked around and counted all the big-name couples. 'No way. There's at least sixteen couples here that we're never going to touch.'

We didn't want to be rude, but we were thinking, *The semi-final? Don't be so silly!* Zipping up our jackets, we ran to find a seat at the back of the arena, where we could watch the rest of the competition. In our seats, I happily counted the numbers as they were being called out for the semi-final. Suddenly I realised that there was only one more number to call and it had to be ours. We were such late entries that we were the last couple to sign up to the championships and our entry number was 350, which was the highest number among the couples remaining from the previous round.

I tugged Ben's arm. 'We're in,' I said excitedly.

He brushed me off. 'Shut up!'

'And couple number 350 . . .' said the announcer.

It really was us! We gasped, unzipped our jackets and ran as fast as we could to get onto the floor. Only, Ben's jacket wouldn't fully unzip. 'I can't get it off!' he said, his voice full of panic.

'Couple number 350!' the announcer said again.

'I'm going to have to go on with my jacket on!' Ben hissed.

He managed to whip it off just as he emerged onto the floor to see everybody on their feet, clapping and cheering. Suddenly we were face to face with the other couples in the semis. Are you kidding us? We're dancing in the same round as these superstars? With dance legends Barbara McColl and Brian Watson on the judging panel?

Darren Hammond, a dancer from South Africa, came up to us and gave us the biggest hug; we looked over to Richard Porter and he gave us a massive grin.

We went out there and jived our hearts out, and the audience gave us a standing ovation. Brimming with excitement, when the cameras came off us at the end I ran up to Richard and jumped on him, even though he had a back injury. Oops!

The judges placed us twelfth in the world and we just couldn't believe it. None of our friends or family had been there to see it, so it almost didn't seem real. There we were, just the two of us, FaceTiming our parents and screaming, 'We just made the semi-finals at the World Championships and came twelfth!'

They couldn't contain their excitement on the other end of the phone. They were jumping about, celebrating like mad; Dad was close to tears; Mum kept shaking her head in disbelief. Ben and I were a couple who didn't have a name; we'd had to work so hard; and now suddenly everyone saw us as contenders – internationally, as well as nationally. It was a huge turnaround. And what a relief for Mum and Dad. All they'd ever wanted was for me to be happy.

What do you do when you've just had the biggest result of your career? We were both really hungry, but after we'd stayed to watch the final all the nearby food outlets were closed, and we had no money anyway, or only enough for a sandwich. So we went to a vending machine, bought two chocolate bars and sat on our hotel bed, still stunned at our result, eating our snacks in a happy daze.

'Here's to winning the title next year,' Ben said, raising his bar of Milka like a glass of wine.

'Cheers to that,' I laughed, toasting him back with my Ritter Sport.

Chapter 6

Sometimes the hardest decisions turn out to be the best ones

L ife is full of decisions. All day long we're making choices. Most of them are minor and don't take up much space in our brains. Coffee or tea? Bath or shower? Orange or pink? But then along come the big decisions, the difficult ones. The I-just-don't-know-what-to-do moments that drive us to distraction because there's no obvious plan to settle on. What then?

Well, one thing I've learned over the years is to take ownership of my decisions, for better or for worse. From my *Strictly* choreography to going public about having Crohn's disease, and whether or not to have chemotherapy, I've realised that it's up to me to take responsibility for the choices I make. That way, if something doesn't work out, I've only got myself to blame. And if it does, great.

Take choreography: on *Strictly Come Dancing*, the professional dancers and their celebrity partners work in collaboration with the show's brilliant team of experts to decide on music, costumes and concepts for each performance. The producers come with ideas and we come with ideas, but they make the overall decisions, because they're planning each show as a balance of types of dances and musical genres.

However, once all that is decided, when it comes to the choreography of a couple routine, it's up to the pros, because that's where our expertise lies. We can get help with it if we want to, or we can create it entirely ourselves – and I prefer to do it myself. Then, if the judges don't like it, or if the audience don't like it, when I go home it's on me, isn't it? And if it goes really well and scores a forty, I own it. Yay!

It sounds like I've got it all worked out, but I haven't, honestly. I'm just like everybody else in having times when I don't know what to do. Life can be really confusing for us all and it's all too easy to be guided by outside influences, especially in this social media era that we live in. Even when it's just your friends and family who are firing opinions and advice at you, it's horrible not being able to make up your mind. The pressure of it can make you feel like your head is going to explode.

That's how it was for me in 2016, when I came up against the most difficult decision I'd ever had to make. My brain was on fire and I had to fight an epic battle with all my conflicting thoughts before I came to realise that I'd known the answer all along.

But it took me a while to get there.

It was the spring of 2016 and all Ben and I could think about was the next British National Dance Championships – 'the Nationals' – coming up in November. There's never total certainty, but after being placed second the year before, this was our best chance yet of becoming champions. Fingers crossed, the lessons, hard work and dedication were about to pay off. We just had to keep going and fix our eyes on the goal.

It was such a big deal. The biggest deal of our lives so far. Winning the Nationals in Blackpool is like being awarded a PhD in Latin dancing. It's the pinnacle in our industry, a title that can never be taken away from you. It makes you eligible to judge competitions, gives you lifelong credit and makes your name forever. You are a 'former British champion' and always will be, and students from all over will want to be taught by you. If we could win the Nationals, our future would be a lot more secure.

There were no guarantees we'd do it, of course. There were so many things that could go wrong: the judges could decide against us; a new partnership might form and come out of nowhere to beat us; we might not dance well on the night; I could have a Crohn's flare-up and be unable to go on . . .

But you can't think about the negative stuff when you're aiming to win. You have to be positive. We're going to make it this time, we kept telling ourselves.

It was like we had blinkers on. We couldn't see anything except our route to success. All our energy was focused in one direction and the closer we came to making our dream real, the more our drive and determination surged. But then, out of the blue, a huge obstacle appeared on the road ahead. Actually, it was more like a mirage, to be accurate, because it was beautiful and dreamlike – and, wow, did it complicate things.

✦

One morning, Jack, one of the producers on *Strictly Come Dancing*, sent me a message saying that the production team were doing some research for the programme. Jack had been following me for a while and asked if I would be interested in having a Skype chat with the production team.

'Course!' I said.

For me, *Strictly Come Dancing* has always been more than just a dance show. It got me through the darkest times of my illness and was a big inspiration in keeping me dancing. So when I jumped on the Skype call, I started chatting away, happily giving them all my feedback, delighted to share my passion for the show. Little did I know they were calling me to suss out my character and personality. I was being interviewed.

A day or two later, Jack rang me. 'Would you be able to come down to London to see us? We'd love to consider you as a professional dancer on the show.'

My mouth dropped open. 'Me? Are you sure?' I stammered.

I was amazed and a bit taken aback. Although I loved *Strictly* with all my heart, my whole mind and energy were focused on winning at Blackpool.

'Do you mean this year?' I asked.

I felt dizzy at the thought of being considered. It was a mix of pleasure, shock and confusion. Did they really mean it? Surely they knew that Ben and I were going all out to win the Nationals later in the year, when *Strictly* would also be broadcast? I couldn't remember if I'd mentioned it to Jack, but I must have, I thought. He would have known about it anyway, surely.

But now my mind went into overdrive and I couldn't help thinking about how my life would change if I got a job on one of the biggest TV shows in the UK. Ben and I could go on holiday somewhere really nice, maybe even move out and get our own place! I started writing a shopping list in my mind, beginning with some nice outfits, pretty dresses and a cosmetics upgrade from No7 to MAC. With my TV earnings, I could splash out at last!

Yet all the while, in the back of my mind, was the sinking feeling that I'd have to turn down any offer they made, if it came to it. *Strictly* weren't reaching out to Ben as well, so how could I abandon our plans to dance at Blackpool and leave him in the lurch? It's every dancer's dream to be crowned a champion in Blackpool and it had been our goal from the day we started dancing together. How could I take that away from him? He had stood by me without a second thought every time a Crohn's flare-up forced me to pull out of a competition or show. Now was my chance to stick by him. But would it be the best decision – for both of us – in the long run?

I asked my family what they thought I should do. 'It's not just Blackpool; it's our dance school,' I said, listing the reasons why doing *Strictly* was out of the question. Ben and I were working towards opening our own dance academy and already had masses of students. How could I walk away from them, as well?

'Just go and meet the show's producers. You never know,' my family said.

I went back to *Strictly*. 'When do you want me to come?'

They weren't wasting any time. 'Is this weekend any good?'

'Oh, no, sorry, I'm with my formation teams at Blackpool.'

They suggested some other dates. 'Sorry, I can't do that date,' I said, and, 'Oh, I can't do that one, either.'

I was stalling because I knew in my heart that it was a dead end. But they must have thought it was a bit weird. I mean, who does that to the BBC?

✦

When it came to it, I decided to leave the British Open Formation Championships early in order to travel to meet them in London. We met up centrally in a gym and Jack introduced me to *Strictly*'s executive producer at the time, Louise – except that I was so wound up with nerves that I didn't catch her job title or realise how important she was.

We sat down for a chat and I started blabbering away, telling them about the weekend in Blackpool and showing them all the pictures of my kids competing in the formation championships. Then we went into one of the dance studios, where I taught Jack a waltz and a cha-cha, and they asked me some questions to camera. It was fun – an interesting experience, if nothing else – but I didn't think anything would come of it.

When it was over, as I was walking out of the gym I passed another dancer, who looked me up and down, as if to say, 'What are you doing here?'

I didn't know what to say. 'I'm thinking the same as you!' I blurted out.

On the train back to Birmingham, I rang my mum, still in disbelief that *Strictly* were even interested in me and had scouted me. When I got home that night, it was the BAFTAs on the telly, and when *Strictly* won, there on the screen, collecting the award, was Louise. 'Oh my goodness, that lady on the telly interviewed me today!' I gasped.

I thought back to how I'd gone in, chatty Amy, babbling away. Then I thought that maybe it was good I hadn't known how important she was, because it probably would have made me a lot more nervous.

Two days later, Jack rang and offered me the chance to become one of the professional dancers on *Strictly Come Dancing*. My dream job, basically – the role I had been longing for ever since I saw the very first episode of the show, when I was fourteen. I'd done it. I'd got there! My lifelong goal was right there in front of my eyes and all I had to do was step forward and take it. What should I do?

Then a horrible thought occurred to me. I hadn't told any of the team about my Crohn's disease. It wasn't that I'd forgotten about it, because obviously I was living with it and managing it every day. But I didn't speak about it with anyone beyond my close family and friends, and I was used to putting it in a box when I went about my professional life. It was a secret, I guess, or as close to one as it possibly could be.

It was hard to imagine a show as massive as *Strictly* being willing to take the risk of me falling ill on live TV. I imagined them saying, 'Oh no, sorry, that changes everything.' But I knew I had to tell them, all the same.

I accepted the job provisionally and when I met up with the production team to go over my contract, it was really difficult to find the words. 'I need to tell you something . . . ' I said, haltingly. Eventually, I just garbled it.

Their expressions didn't change. 'Oh, that's fine,' they said. 'Just make sure you put it down on the insurance form. And let us know if there's anything we can do to help.'

And that was that. I couldn't believe it. After all the heartache I'd been through with my Crohn's over the years, they didn't think it was an issue.

'So you're not worried about it?' I asked.

'Darling, if you can go on the dance floor and be the dancer you are, Crohn's disease isn't going to get in the way. We've watched you dance and do so well. Why would we worry?'

Wow, they accept it! I thought. This is amazing.

Then I explained about Blackpool. 'I can't take this moment away from Ben, our coach, our families . . .'

They understood. They said they would maybe try to find a way for me to have that weekend in November off, and my heart leaped. It wouldn't be ideal, because doing *Strictly* would reduce my practice time with Ben down to almost nothing, but maybe we could make it work.

✦

What I didn't know was that protocol set by the British Dance Council at the time ruled me out of taking part in an amateur competition if I was working as a professional dancer. Since I would be dancing in the amateur section of the Nationals, this was a problem. (There's very little difference in standard between amateur and professional, but you tend not to go professional until later in your career, unless you have to.) When I challenged the protocol, I was advised that even if I was treated as a special case and the Council waived their usual rules for me, the system wouldn't like it and the judges at the Nationals might go against me. 'You've always done things the right way. You've got a great reputation. Don't ruin it now,' I was told.

I had to make a choice between the Nationals and *Strictly*. I phoned Philip and Carol, and Mum and Dad, and talked it through. 'I don't know what to do!' I said, in a panic.

I had advice coming from everywhere. I had people on *Strictly* calling and saying, 'Why are you hesitating? You'll never get this opportunity again,' and others saying, 'Do Blackpool! You've been wanting to win the finals at Blackpool all your life!'

I had to think so hard about it. But something in my heart was saying that it was the wrong time for *Strictly*. Deep down I knew I wouldn't be able to live with myself if I took away Ben's chances of winning at Blackpool. It takes years to build up a partnership, so he couldn't have danced it with anyone else.

And it wasn't just about Ben – I didn't know if I was going to like TV, or if I would be liked or wanted there. Was I going to take away everything from Ben to be selfish and dive into a world I knew nothing about? And yet how could I not? How could I throw away such an amazing opportunity?

I talked it over with Ben and we tried to weigh up the pros and cons. Ultimately, it was up to me. 'I'll stand by you, no matter what you decide,' Ben said.

That's Ben. Generous and unselfish to the last. My partner and my love, who I'd worked so hard with, who had stood by me through so many Crohn's flare-ups. He had never given up hope on me. How could I turn around and throw all that in his face?

I had to be the one to make the decision, because then I couldn't blame anybody else for what happened next. It was on me. I kept going back and forward in my mind. How could I take the *Strictly* job? How could I *not* take it? I didn't make up my mind until the very last minute and I'm sorry for the anguish that must have caused Ben, even though he knew I had both our interests at heart. If I became a dancer on *Strictly*, we would both benefit. If I didn't, we would have to go on running ourselves ragged just getting by until the Nationals in November. And even then, there were no guarantees.

✦

The day came when I had to make my decision. That morning, I woke up with a totally clear mind. I was going to go with what my gut was telling me and make the choice I could live with for the rest of my life, out of love for my partner and for the whole dancing world.

I rang up *Strictly* to let them know. But I was so upset that I couldn't speak and had to hang up. I sent an email instead. I poured my heart into it. 'Dear the entire *Strictly* family,' I wrote, 'I'm truly sorry for any inconvenience I have caused and for being so emotional on the phone earlier. This has been the hardest decision I've ever had to make . . . I am truly devastated and upset to be unable to be part of *Strictly* this year.'

I was the first ever professional dancer to turn *Strictly* down and I wanted them to know how much I hated doing it. But I had no idea if my words were falling on deaf ears.

'I can't thank you all enough for the time and opportunity you gave me,' I wrote, and continued:

> It would have been amazing and a dream come true if it was possible for me to do both – compete with Ben and be part of the *Strictly* family. I feel I owe it to Ben and my coaches to finish my amateur career with him. We've invested so much time, dreams, belief and loyalty in our partnership. I hope this shows that if I'm

ever lucky enough to be part of *Strictly* in the future, I would give the show my entire commitment and loyalty.

Ben and I have worked for many years towards the next couple of months of competitions. Both my dreams came at the very same time, the British Championships and *Strictly Come Dancing*. I tried my best to be loyal, not selfish, and do the right thing.

Over the past few months, the team has simply felt like a dream team. I really do hope I get the opportunity to one day experience and be part of the show. I would like to take this opportunity to thank everyone for being so kind and supportive these last few months. No wonder the show is so successful with the team you have. I wish you all, from the bottom of my heart, the best of luck. Not that you need it with the series. I'll be watching and supporting all the way. Thank you again, it's still and always will be a dream of mine to work with *Strictly* in the future and I'm truly devastated it hasn't worked out this year.

The exec emailed me back to say how disappointed she was to receive my email, but that she understood my reasons, appreciated that it hadn't been an easy decision and said how impressed the team had been with me. 'I am confident that you would have enjoyed being part of the *Strictly* family,' she wrote, and wished me good luck for the Nationals. 'Do keep in touch,' she added.

And just like that, my *Strictly* dreams went up in a puff of smoke. What made it doubly hard was knowing that the pressure was even greater now on us to win the Nationals, because I'd given up *Strictly* so that I could compete there with Ben. I couldn't bear to think how much regret I'd feel if we didn't win, having made such a huge sacrifice. And where would we be then?

Stop! I told myself, when my thoughts started spiralling. Be positive. We *will* win.

I knew I couldn't control what happened on the night. All I could do was put in the work and stay upbeat.

Before we knew it, the Nationals were upon us. It's a three-day event and the amateur competition is held on the last day. Ben and I watched the first two days in the ballroom with my sister, Rebecca, and Ben's best friend, Ian, who looked after us throughout the competition. We were super stressed and they did everything to keep us calm – Rebecca with me and Ian with Ben, including keeping us apart so that we didn't make each other even more nervous. Ben and I literally met up to dance.

Rebecca had been my rock at the Nationals every year. She did practically everything for me, except compete for me: she'd be up for hours the night before, gluing gems on my dance shoes and dance dress; she fetched me cups of coffee and water; she laid out my make-up and helped me with my hair.

This time, I tried to get as much sleep as I could the night before the competition, but so much is on your mind, along with the excitement of wanting to dance. I put on another layer of tan before I went to bed. Rebecca and I double-checked that I had everything I needed. We set it all out for the next day, so that there was no stress when I was getting ready. Everything had to go smoothly. There couldn't be any bumps in the road.

In the morning, Ben and I went to practise. Afterwards, Rebecca helped me get ready for the evening. She knew how to keep our hotel room very chilled – that's probably her experience as a midwife kicking in. I was incredibly jittery and she was a brilliant support and calming influence.

If I had the choice, I would have wanted Rebecca at every competition I danced in – and she was at a lot of them, to be fair. She loved watching us compete. Being a dancer herself, she would tell me when she thought we'd danced well or badly, or when we were hard done by. She was very honest, at the same time championing me and saying, 'You can do this.' She was my number one fan and whenever I doubted myself she believed in me.

When she moved to Australia at the end of 2015, I waved her off on the bus, yelling, 'You've got to come back for Blackpool!'

And here she was.

As the minutes counted down to the start of the competition, it felt reassuring to know that I had my family with me, despite my fluttering heart. My mum and dad were there, of course, my lifelong supporters. I desperately wanted them to know how grateful I was to them for believing in me, even when at times I think they would have preferred me to do anything except dance. They'd put up with so much over the years – so much worry, mostly, but also a lot of expense, driving, rearranging and rushing around for me – as well as all those days and nights spent by my hospital bed, on top of everything else. They had guided me, pushed me and loved me throughout my dancing journey. So, more than anything, I wanted to make them proud tonight.

I was glad that Lloyd was there, too – my quiet, sensitive, super-intelligent, fun brother – with his lovely wife, Holly. Bless him, Lloyd sacrificed the most out of the three of us, growing up. He didn't ever moan about the fact that Rebecca and I were always dancing, even when he was dragged along to Blackpool to watch. I can't imagine how hard it must have been for a teenage boy to be surrounded by under-12s dancing in sparkly costumes over the Easter weekend, when all he really wanted to do was go surfing in Cornwall. Yet he was always supportive, even though we went to my granddad's static caravan less and less as the dancing took off.

Then there were Carol and Philip Perry, my second mum and dad, who supported my dancing in every way they could. They didn't have to; it wasn't as if they were living out their dreams through me. They were Welsh champions, they'd won *Come Dancing,* the weekly TV dance contest that ran from 1950 to 1998 and inspired *Strictly* – and their children and grandchildren went on to be champions, as well. But still they supported me and showed me love during my darkest times: when I collapsed and was rushed to hospital; when I was turned down again and again during tryouts with boys who may not have been comfortable with the fact that I had a chronic illness. Carol and Philip were my mentors, but they were also incredibly kind to me; I was so happy they'd be cheering me on now for the biggest challenge of my dancing career.

Everyone important was there to watch our big moment. Well, everyone except Richard Porter, who was in LA. But we could hardly expect him to fly halfway across the world just to see us dance, could we?

I tried to calm my nerves by looking at it another way. *I've been on a really steep learning curve*, I thought. *And it has helped shape the person I am today. So maybe that's enough? Maybe it's not the end of the world if we don't win?*

Over the previous two years, I'd learned so much – the hardship and resilience, respect and humility. And I'd had the most amazing dance lessons that would enable me to go on and be an excellent dance teacher myself. So I knew that, whatever the outcome, the time I'd spent and the sacrifices I'd made would not go to waste. And if I hadn't given myself a shot at becoming a top-level dancer – if I hadn't put in all of those hours of training – I would have always thought, *What if?*

✦

I felt under so much pressure as we went out onto the dance floor for our first routines. The ballroom was packed, every seat filled, and the roar of the crowd was deafening. Richard had trained us not to get sucked into the atmosphere, or into thinking about the competition or the judges, but I knew that today I had to dance the very best I could and give it everything, every inch of my body. I looked over at Rebecca, who smiled and pointed at the heart locket around her neck. My nan had bought us each a heart locket when we were babies and Rebecca always wears hers for special days, like the day of her university interview, when she picked up her A-level results and when she did her driving test. And there she was now, proudly wearing it for my big moment.

Just then, I saw Richard Porter walking towards me. I felt a jolt of surprise. 'What's he doing here?' Ben said.

It turned out that Richard had flown all the way from Los Angeles just to see us dance. Wow! It heightened the emotion to know he cared so much; that he was mindful of how much we had sacrificed and what I'd gone through with my health. But it also put the fear in us, if I'm honest, because impressing Richard was so important to us.

He wasn't there to smile and clap us on, either. He was our coach to the end; he didn't let up. After the semi-final, he came over to me during my dress change. Brad had designed a beautiful black dress for me to wear for the first few rounds and now, for the final, I was changing into a white dress completely covered in diamanté with diamanté-encrusted white shoes. I was hurrying because there wasn't much time between the semi and the final, but he stood in front of me and stopped me in my tracks.

'If we don't win tonight, it'll be your fault,' he said angrily.

'OK,' I said meekly.

My dad came over, with a look of concern on his face. 'What did Richard just say?' he asked.

I was still in shock, trying to absorb Richard's words. 'It's fine!' I murmured.

Richard knew how to press our buttons. I was dancing well, but he just wanted a little bit more fire in my belly for that final.

And I guess it worked, because I went out onto the dance floor and gave every last ounce of the best of me, making sure I focused on the job in hand with no attachment to thoughts or feelings. There was no thinking, *This feels good*, or, *We're winning*. The aim wasn't simply to win, anyway. You want to be remembered forever, to create magic moments for everybody watching.

As we came off the floor, I thought, *I hope that was enough.* As you're one of six couples on the floor dancing at the same time, you can't watch your fellow competitors and really have no idea how you've done.

We waited anxiously for the results, our hearts beating furiously. 'In first place, from Dudley . . . ' came the announcer's voice, 'Amy Dowden and Ben Jones!'

Ben and I were the first all-British pair to win the Amateur Latin category of the Nationals in over twenty years. And I have to say that it doesn't get better than winning the British National Dance Championships with the person you love most in the world. It was the biggest achievement of both our lives and we got to share it.

Was it the right decision to turn down *Strictly Come Dancing*? Yes, I truly believe it was. It's actually simple: when it comes to the important choices in life, you've just got to do the right thing. Otherwise, you may end up regretting it for your whole life to come.

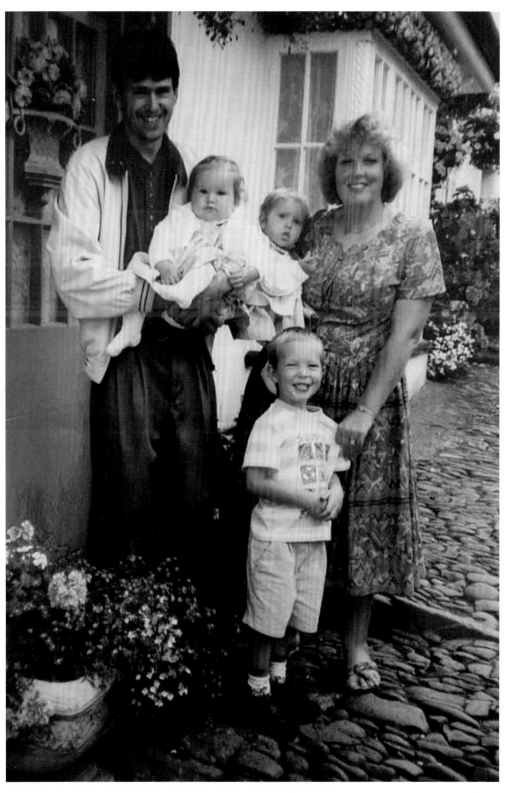

An early photo of all five of us – Dad holding Rebecca, and Mum with me and a beaming Lloyd.

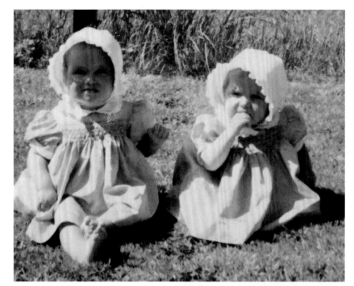

Rebecca and me as babies – very cute, though I suspect those hats make us look more angelic than we were!

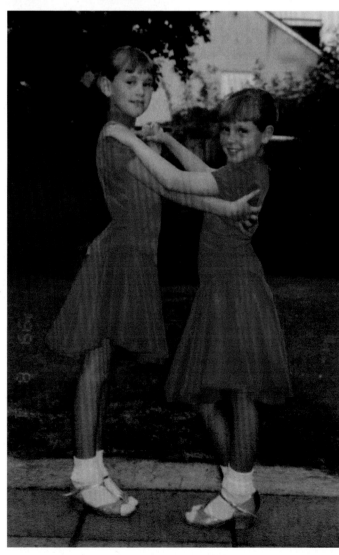

Here we are in our first dance outfits – red satin dresses with full skirts and dance shoes that were a gift from gramps. I still have those gold Cuban heels.

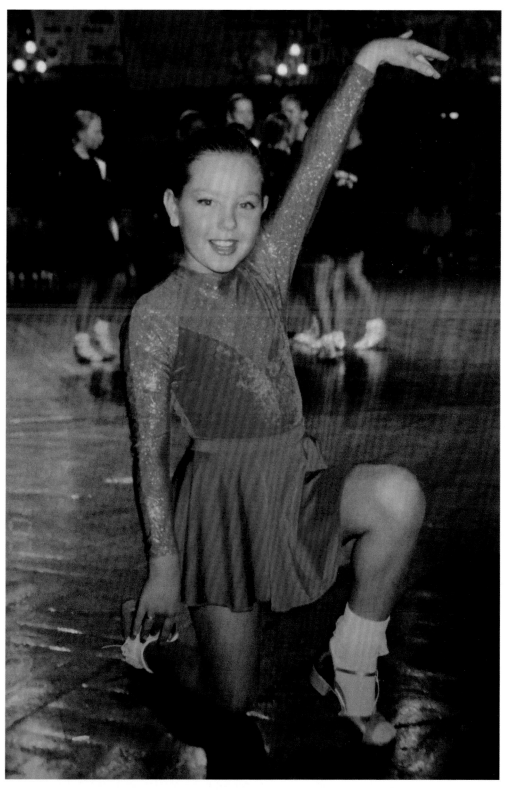

Here I am, age eight, at the Blackpool Tower ballroom for the first time and obviously loving it.

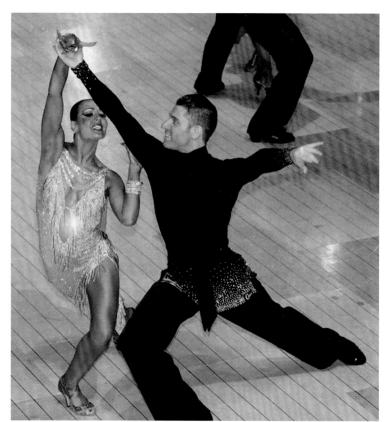

Me and Ben competing at Blackpool in late spring 2015, in the zone, just loving the dancing.

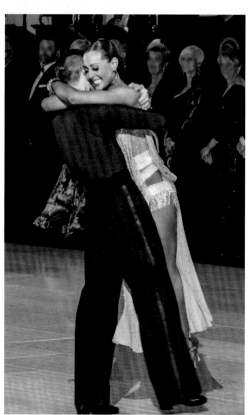

Being awarded second place at the 'Nationals' in November 2015 blew us away. I screamed and Ben cried with joy and relief!

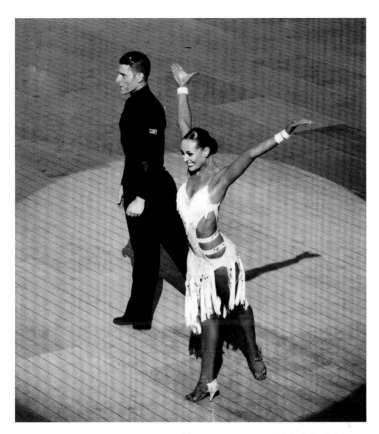

The 'Nationals' at Blackpool, November 2016. I'd given up the offer of joining *Strictly* to compete so we gave it everything we had, and it worked! Finally, we were champions.

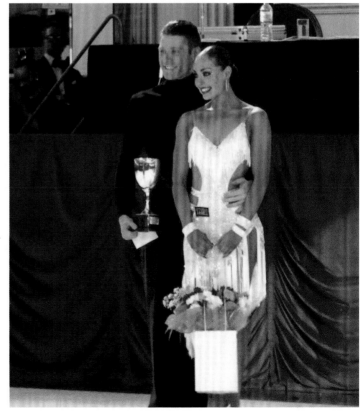

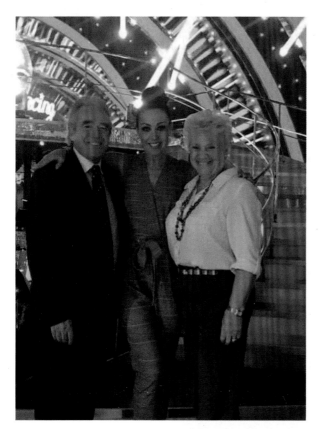

At *Strictly* with dance teachers Carol and Philip Perry, my second mum and dad, who have supported my dancing in every way they could.

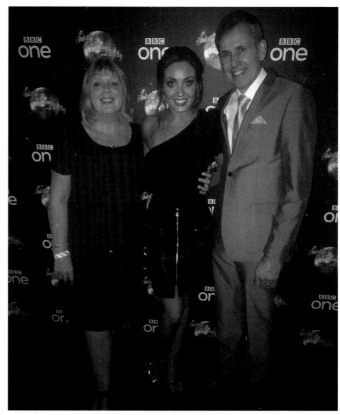

At *Strictly* with my parents in 2018. They were clearly thrilled to be there.

At the *Strictly* final in 2023. I had broken my foot and had a blood clot on my lung, but I was lucky enough to perform a lovely fan dance in the opening number.

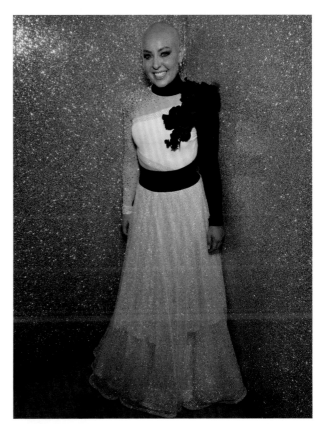

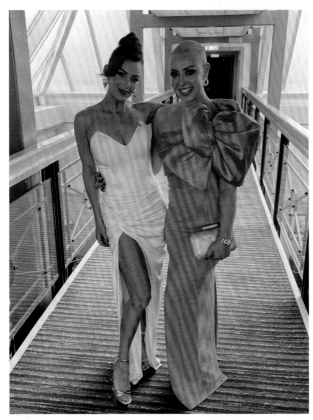

With one of my best friends, Dianne Buswell, at the Pride of Britain awards in 2023. It was the first time I appeared on TV without a wig.

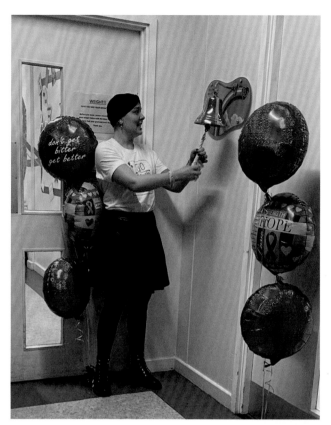

A proud moment ringing the bell to signify my final chemo treatment. I felt such relief to be at that point and so thankful to the oncology team at the Sheldon Unit.

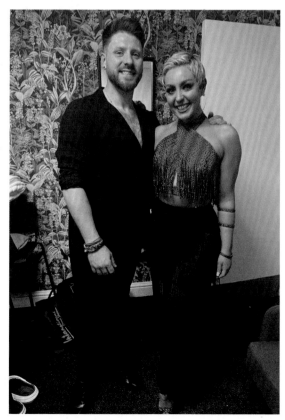

My first dance show with Ben since my cancer diagnosis. It felt amazing to be back where I belong.

Chapter 7

Don't let fear and insecurity hold you back

W hat happens when your biggest dream turns into a nightmare? When you get what you've always wanted, only to find you don't want it any more – in fact, you feel like running away from it as fast as your legs will carry you?

If you've ever had a crisis of confidence, you'll know how shaky it can make you feel. When it happened to me, my childhood dream had just come true and I didn't know how to cope. It sounds like a mixed-up situation, I know. But something deep down was telling me that I wasn't good enough to achieve my goal, and that others deserved it more because they were better than me.

I shouldn't be here! I thought. Not me, not Amy from Wales.

It all started just after the fourteenth series of *Strictly* ended – the series that I had turned down in order to enter the Nationals with Ben. It was a week or so after Ore Oduba and Joanne Clifton won the *Strictly* glitter ball and I emailed the *Strictly* production team to say what a brilliant series it had been. I guess I wanted them to know that my love and passion for the show were as strong as ever.

'Hi, Amy. It was lovely to hear from you, and congratulations on winning the British championships,' came the reply. 'We gave you a big cheer when we heard you had done so well, and it was thoroughly well deserved. Thanks for your kind words about the series. We're all very proud of it, but we now have our feet firmly back on the ground as we gear up again for the next series. When do you think you'll turn professional? And what are your plans for next year?'

My heart skipped a beat when I read their words. They were asking about my future as a professional dancer! Did that mean they were still considering me for the show? After the agony and difficulty of what had happened the year before, I didn't dare ask; I could only hope.

And then I heard nothing from them.

✦

In early 2017, Ben and I were busier than ever. Now that we were the British champions – at last! – we were in demand to dance in shows, demonstrations and competitions all over the UK and internationally, anything from an event at a dance school in London or a dinner dance in Cardiff, to a championship ball in California. But, for us, the most important date on our calendar was the British Open Championships in Blackpool in May, which is the biggest ballroom and Latin American dancing competition in the world. When you're the British champions, this is obviously the one competition you can't miss – and what made it even more important was knowing it would be our last amateur competition before turning professional.

For me, there was an added pull, too. I had a strong feeling that the team from *Strictly* would be there to scout dancers.

More than anything, I wanted to try to impress them all over again.

The day of the British Open arrived. Ben and I reached the quarter-finals, the top twenty-four couples in the world, and we were the last British pair left in the competition. It was everything we had hoped for and we were feeling good. The Blackpool Winter Gardens were absolutely packed. Even up in the gods, people were standing on spotlights and hanging over balconies to get a view of the last stages of the Open.

I scoured the audience to see if I could spot any members of the *Strictly* production team just before Ben and I went on to dance the cha-cha. Behind a pillar I saw the executive producer and two of the producers, and we made eye contact. The atmosphere was electric, everybody was clapping . . . and I waved to them.

Oh no. How embarrassing! Like, who does that? If my students waved at someone in a competition I'd tell them off. I was mortified at myself. But now I had to focus. I knew I had to dance my heart out. I had to dance the best I'd ever danced, for the *Strictly* team to see. I went out onto the dance floor and gave it my all, and when we came off, I ran around the building to check if they were still there. They weren't. They'd gone. I was gutted that I hadn't got to speak to them.

I've missed my chance, I thought.

Two days later, I was teaching dance classes in a special needs school when I missed four phone calls in a row. You can't answer the phone when you're in school and my heart sank as I left the building, because I recognised the *Strictly* phone number.

I ran to my car. The phone rang again. 'Are you somewhere on your own?' said the voice of one of the producers.

'Yes, I'm in my car,' I replied breathlessly, my heart thumping.

'Is this a good year, Amy?' she asked. 'Would you like to join *Strictly*?'

I screamed and burst into tears. After all that had happened, I just couldn't believe it. 'Oh, yes, please!' I kept saying.

I raced home in a total fluster, desperate to tell Ben the good news. Only, how would he react? If I went off to join *Strictly*, our competing days would be over. Plus, Ben and I had done everything together for the past six years and this would mean having a lot of time apart. It wasn't going to be easy. And yet it felt like the best news ever and I couldn't wait to share it.

By the time I got back, I looked so overwrought that Ben thought I'd been in a car accident, or that something had happened to my granddad, who was ill at the time.

'What is it?' he asked worriedly.

I burst out laughing. 'I've got *Strictly*!' I yelled.

If Ben was sad about what it meant for our competing career, he didn't show it. Like me, he thought I'd missed my chance, so he was elated for me now. He was jumping for joy. 'But we can't tell anybody,' I warned. 'We're not doing the press release for a couple of months yet!'

He frowned. 'Not even your mum and dad? Or mine?'

Thankfully, I was allowed to tell my parents, because I wouldn't have been able to keep it a secret from them. I rang my mum, who was still at work, and she cried with happiness right there, in the office. 'Well done, Amy!' she kept saying. 'You deserve it. You've worked so hard.'

Then I rang my dad, who was working on a job in someone's house. 'Dad, I'm gonna be the first Welsh professional on *Strictly*!'

My dad also burst into tears! And then he had to wipe his eyes and go back to his job like everything was normal. A few minutes later, a text came through from him, saying that he just wanted to shout it from the rooftops, and he wished his mum was alive because she'd be so proud, and the best thing he'd ever done was play the triangle at a school concert, and even then he had to wait for someone to nod at him before he knew when to bang it . . . and that just made him extra proud of me!

My only sadness was that my granddad had dementia by then and although he was around for my first few years at *Strictly*, he never truly understood that I was one of the show's dancers. He would have been so proud and so happy if he had. Gramps, as we all called him, loved it when any of us did well at something. Many years earlier, when I'd gone round to his house after school to show him a trophy I'd won, he'd insisted on knocking next door to show it to the neighbours. And when he drove me home, he knocked at our next door, too. 'Look what she's won!' he said, beaming with pride. 'Isn't she brilliant?'

I told Rebecca and my brother Lloyd my news, but otherwise we kept it quiet, and then Ben and I went out to America to train with Richard, as no matter where you are in your career, you want to keep on learning and improving, and we were about to turn professional. We took Phillip and Carol's grandson, also called Lloyd, with us – Lloyd is a talented young dancer and he'd started having lessons with Richard a few months earlier. As he was too young to be in Los Angeles alone, Ben and I used to act as his responsible adults while we were there.

We had adjoining hotel rooms on this trip and the morning of the announcement, Lloyd came bounding into our room, waving his phone. 'It says on the BBC website that you're joining *Strictly*. Is it true?'

'Yes, Lloyd,' I laughed. 'It's on the BBC news.'

'No way!' he yelled.

It was mad how many messages flooded in that day as I lay on my hotel bed in LA, resting between lessons with Richard. And mega exciting the number of followers I was getting on Instagram, especially pro dancers like Gorka Márquez. I reached out to Nadiya Bychkova and Dianne Buswell, who were joining the show as well, and then Oti Mabuse messaged me, saying, 'Congratulations! Can't wait to meet you and work with you.'

'Wow! Oti Mabuse has messaged me!' I screeched.

In the middle of all this, the *Sun* newspaper rang me. 'We just want to ask you what your relationship status is, Amy.'

I put my hand over the receiver. 'What do I say?' I asked Ben.

We'd never actually told anybody we were in a relationship. Everyone knew; they just didn't ask.

'What do you want to say?'

'Shall I just tell them?'

'Yeah,' he laughed.

I took my hand away from my phone. 'I'm in a relation-ship,' I told the reporter.

When I got back to the UK, the kids at our dance school were screaming with excitement that their teacher was going to be on *Strictly*. When they'd calmed down, their curiosity took over. 'The newspaper says you have a boyfriend. Who is it?' they asked.

'It's Ben,' I said.

They squealed in surprise. 'Ben! Really?' It was so funny, because their mums knew, everybody knew, but they had no idea.

'It was perfectly clear,' my parents said. 'You didn't need to tell anybody. We all knew.'

Apparently, Ben's dad had been saying to my dad, 'Yes, they're definitely together.'

And all the while, we thought we were fooling everybody.

Through all this excitement, Ben and I kept our feet on the ground, working hard, even up to and over the weekend before I started *Strictly* on the Monday, when we competed in our first professional UK championships. Of course, we weren't expecting miracles from our first performance in the professional dance arena. Normally, when you go up to the pro division, you'll just about make the final if you're lucky, and we thought we might get to sixth place. But we did so much better than expected. We came second and nearly won. It was a massive surprise and I think a lot of pros in the industry were thinking, *Why are you going off to* Strictly *when you've got this?*

This very unexpected result planted a seed of doubt in my mind – and I was so conscious of what Ben was giving up for me that I had that guilt as well. I knew how sad he must be that his competing days were coming to an end because of me. Of course, I wouldn't have held him back if he'd wanted to start a new partnership, but I knew it wasn't on his radar. I was his dance partner; we still wanted to dance together and had big plans to grow our newly founded dance school. And starting a new partnership is not an easy thing to do – you're at the back of the pack once more, you've got to do all that work again together, and it takes years. And we didn't know how I was going to find *Strictly*. Was I going to love it? Was I going to be asked back? We wanted to leave the door open in case we wanted to return to competing.

My thoughts turned to the coming week and what was in store for me at the *Strictly Come Dancing* rehearsals, and my nerves began to kick in big time. Would I fit in? Would anyone like me? Was I a good enough dancer?

By the morning of my first day, I was in a state of turmoil. My childhood dream had finally come true and I was scared out of my mind. For six years, I'd only ever danced with Ben. It was just me and him: we lived together, taught together, competed together and practised together every day. Ben was my safety blanket for all that time, and now he was gone and I was going into the room alone.

I got up at dawn to get ready and arrived at the BBC studios an hour and a half early. Taking a deep breath, I stepped into a brand new world. And this new world was filled with amazing, expressive dancers who all had big personalities to match their talent. These were people I really looked up to and they all seemed to know each other, but I was so nervous I couldn't say a word to any of them. There I was, tiptoeing in unnoticed, totally in awe of everyone, little Amy from Wales, hoping to be accepted.

Who did I think I was?

I kept a smile on my face but felt myself shrink inside as I looked around the room. The other dancers were radiating confidence, but I felt so small, so insignificant. It was daunting to think that soon I would be dancing with some of these boys, in couples. I was only used to dancing with Ben! What if they didn't like my style of dancing?

I'm not good enough to be here! I thought. I must have been mad to think I was.

I tried to stay in the background all morning and sat on my own at lunchtime, feeling overwhelmed. *This is awful*, I thought. *Everyone else is being so sociable, but I'm not fitting in at all. No one likes me!*

Kevin Clifton came over and sat with me. I guessed that he'd come to give me words of encouragement and support, but his presence made me feel uncomfortable. 'Remember,' he said, 'the production team wanted you on the show because they love you and they love your dancing.'

'Mmm, mm,' I replied, nodding and smiling, too shy to actually say anything to this guy who had been my absolute idol when I was a kid.

I could tell he was worried that I wasn't chatting, because you've got to be a big personality to be on the show.

'You can talk to me anytime, you know,' he went on. 'Anytime at all. Just believe in yourself, Amy. They want you for you, and they want you to be yourself.'

I nodded again. 'Mmm.'

What I love about Kevin is that he champions everybody. If someone has done a great dance or a brilliant piece of choreography on the show, he will tell them, even to this day. But just then I was trapped in my own head, thinking, *Why am I here? Have I made the right decision? Should I just stick to pro dancing with Ben?*

By the time I left rehearsals that day, I was in a total state. I called Ben and begged him to come and pick me up. 'I can't do it,' I told him. 'It's not how I thought it would be. It's not for me. I'm going to quit. Please take me home.'

'It'll get better,' he said. 'Of course the first day was nerve-racking. You need to give it at least a week before you make a decision.'

'Wha—? No, please, Ben, I can't!'

I hung up and rang my friend Katie, who works with us at our dance school. I cried my eyes out down the phone to her, while sitting on a bench at Waterloo station. 'Ben won't come and get me. Will you?'

'I've just spoken to Ben, Amy,' she said. 'He's right, isn't he? You should try it for at least a week.'

I was staying with my Auntie Carole, who lives in London, and she came and met me at Waterloo. She sat down and comforted me as I sobbed my heart out to her. 'I'm not good enough. I can't do it,' I kept saying, over and over.

It seemed to me that the other new dancers were much more confident than I was: Nadiya, steely and self-assured, and Dianne, who has this bubbly Australian personality. Dianne wasn't even particularly aware of *Strictly* before they asked her to join and she found it all great fun. Me, though,

I was tongue-tied. I grew up watching *Strictly* on telly and knew what a big deal it was. At the same time, I'd had this vision of the show since I was a teenage girl and I didn't want it to be destroyed.

Three days in, the production team took us all out for a night to 'toast the series'. They do it every year and it's a sort of get-to-know-you evening where they tell you about their plans for the upcoming *Strictly* season. I think it really helped with my nerves to be out with everyone off-duty. I felt I could relax and be myself a bit more – and as I got to know everyone a bit better, a change came over me. I began to believe in myself and feel part of it.

'You were meant to do the show last year, weren't you?' people kept saying.

'You know about that, do you?' I replied.

'Yeah, and we think you're amazing!'

I was still a bit dazed. At one point, Aljaž Škorjanec was chatting away to me; at another, Oti was drawing me out of my shell.

'Where are you living?' Oti asked me.

'I'm looking for a place, but until I find somewhere I'm staying with my aunt,' I explained.

'I need someone to live with,' she yelped. 'I've got a free bedroom at my place. Come and live with me!'

I came away from that night with a big smile on my face. When I got back to my auntie's house, I was feeling so much lighter and happier. 'How was it? Are you feeling better now?' she asked.

I threw myself into her arms. 'I loved it!' I said, and she was very relieved to hear it.

I realised that it was my fault the first few days hadn't gone well. I should have gone in and opened up to people, if only to admit how nervous and vulnerable I felt to be in London, starting on *Strictly* without Ben. I knew now that they would have understood and offered their support. Everything else would have followed.

The next morning, Oti sent me a FaceTime video request and photos with captions saying, 'See? This is where you'll live.'

Oh, she means it! I thought, flushing with pleasure.

After that, I was in my element, going into work every day and learning new routines, thrilled to be collaborating with the world's best choreographers and my new friends. Then, before I knew it, the celebrities started being announced! It was a very exciting period, not just for me, but for my family as well.

Gorka jokes that, because I didn't talk in the first week of rehearsals, they sent me off for video and media training to help me feel more at ease on and off camera, even though I didn't need it. 'Send her back!' he often says, because since then I haven't shut up and now I'm the chattiest pro (although only outside rehearsals). 'We want the silent Amy back!'

I realised that Ben had been right, as usual. I had to have that week to get used to things and then I began to accept that I was worthy of my place on *Strictly Come Dancing*.

When I was paired with Kevin during rehearsals one day, I was finally brave enough to tell him how much I'd always looked up to him. 'I absolutely loved watching you when I was a kid! You were my dancing hero. You inspired me,' I told him.

Kevin just laughed it off, but Claudia Winkelman teases me about it to this day. I don't mind; yes, I was a super-fan once, but I'm now really good friends with Kevin and his sister Jo.

✦

Soon my friends and family were asking, 'Who's your celebrity partner? You must know who it is. Tell us! We won't tell anyone.'

'I don't know, I honestly don't,' I protested.

My parents came up for the first show and saw for themselves that it's a genuinely surprising moment when our partners are revealed. Although, by the time it got down to Oti, Katya and me – the last three girls left – I was pretty sure I'd be paired with Brian Conley.

Why? Well, the production team take a lot of care when it comes to matching people and they're really good at it. Yes, they look at your height, but it's mainly decided by personality – and we're all so different. The producers know us pros inside out, and know which of us are firm in training, the softies and the ones who are a bit more relaxed. If someone's looking for creativity and great teaching, that's a Katya student – she can take an absolute beginner all the way; if they're looking for a partner who is wild, wacky, young at heart, carefree and loves TikTok and Instagram, that's Dianne. She's such a big personality and very caring, so when someone young like Bobby Brazier comes on, the obvious pairing for him would be Dianne. Then you've got Luba Mushtuk and Nadiya Bychkova, who are quieter and more reserved, and very sexy, so they're maybe better suited to being matched with someone older.

There is a day dedicated to meeting the celebrities and that's when the production team can see which personalities connect. Early on, Brian Conley came up to me and said something funny, and I started rolling around laughing. I got his sense of humour instantly and, being a comedian, he liked that – especially when I started to complain that my belly ached from laughing. Then, when we were learning a group dance and he was struggling with the steps, I helped him out and he soon got the hang of it.

After the rehearsal, he went straight up to the producers and said, 'I'd like Amy as my partner, please.'

They could already see how well we were getting on. We didn't stop giggling, we felt comfortable around each other, and I was helping him with his routines ... They saw the connection and how it would work well on the show. And they were right in thinking that Brian would be the perfect first partner for me. As well as being a comedian, he's an actor, TV presenter, singer and all-round entertainer, with decades of TV experience and knowledge about this whole new world that I'd only just entered. He gave me confidence.

So I taught Brian dancing and he showed me how to be on camera, how to find the red light and to do TV interviews. He was absolutely brilliant for me. Not the best dancer, but I've never laughed so much in my life as I did with Brian, and he was kind and encouraging, too.

I'll never forget the first time we danced live on *Strictly*. I was all over the place beforehand. I couldn't believe I was going to be making my entrance walking down those world-famous stairs. All those years I'd watched in awe as professional dancers took those stairs with their partners! I was so emotional that I kept having moments where I just wanted to burst into tears. Poor Lisa Armstrong, who was doing my make-up, had to redo my face several times.

'Amy! Don't cry!' she pleaded, every time she saw my eyes start filling with tears again.

In the end, Brian had to have a word and give me some tough love. 'Amy, there's an audience out there – and your family, and the kids at home – who can't wait to see you dancing,' he said. 'Come on, pull yourself together. Get your dancing shoes on, get your dancing head on, and go out there and dance.'

I waited backstage for my mum and dad to come through to their seats. They said it was quite a shock to see me jump out of the shadows and call them over. 'Mum! Dad! I'm so nervous!'

'You're going to be amazing,' they said, although they felt as nervous as I did.

I was overwhelmed by the feeling that I didn't want to let anybody down. After all, I'd brought my competitive career to a halt and stopped dancing with Ben for this. *Strictly* is not just the biggest entertainment show in our country – it's the biggest dance show worldwide, even up against all the other versions of the show in other countries. Every dancer wants to win the British version of *Strictly* – and don't I know it! I've watched it and loved it since I was a girl.

I also wondered, *What if the nation doesn't like me?*

There I was, about to step out and dance on television, watched by all my friends, my family and the kids I taught at my dance school, not to mention millions of people I'd never met. I was going to chat with Tess and Claudia on TV, and face the judges – it was a lot to take in. I was a nervous wreck. Yet when the curtain opened and I walked down the *Strictly* stairs with Brian, I couldn't help breaking into a grin. *Wow, I'm here!* I thought.

Then we danced and I just loved it. I felt the rush of adrenalin and instantly knew: this is where I belong. I'm not going back to the competing world. This is me.

It's just so joyful being on *Strictly*. Yes, you're competing and you want the best for your celebrity, but even if you get sent home, you're still part of an incredible team and get to go back every week. It's upsetting when your celebrity has been eliminated, but the recompense is being in such a lovely environment for the rest of the series.

Competitions are also rewarding, but the good results are far and few between, and often you work really hard for very little return. You pay to enter a competition, you pay for your dress and travel, you do your own hair and make-up; it's tough and expensive and then, when you don't get the result you want, it's total heartache. And you have to pick yourself up again. Even if you win in the Nationals in Blackpool, the pinnacle of competitions, the prize money barely covers the cost of your hotel room. You're doing it purely for the love of dancing and competing. At *Strictly*, you get to do everything you love in one bundle: choreograph, teach (I love teaching!) and perform. You get all the glitz and the glam – the best hair and make-up team making you look good, your amazing dresses made to measure – and you're in this TV family that wrap themselves around you. Everyone is supporting and helping each other. It's very different from being in competition. There is literally nothing not to love. And then, to top it all off, you're going to be paid for it!

✦

Until I joined *Strictly*, Ben and I hadn't a penny to our names. In fact, we were in debt from paying for our dance lessons in Los Angeles. But now we were able to do something we'd always wanted to do and invest in own dance academy with its own premises. While we'd started a dance school a couple of years earlier, we'd been teaching out of church halls and other venues. Now we had a chance to really establish ourselves. 'Let's get our own place!' we agreed.

We rented an industrial unit and I invested all my *Strictly* earnings into turning it into a dance studio. It was full-on hard work and Ben's family were an amazing help, from doing the books to painting the walls. Our existing students' parents chipped in as well to help out. We were really lucky the way our community came together for us. Brian Conley even helped us by becoming a patron, because he knew how much the academy meant to us.

Every time I visited our new academy, I'd walk in and think, I can't believe this is ours! It really felt like we'd made it, at last. Ben was rushed off his feet sorting everything out while I was away, on top of his already busy teaching schedule. We'd had to become quite independent after I joined *Strictly*. Ben had to live on his own for a couple of months of the year and there's not many people who could cope with their partner being away for so long, or who would be happy for her to live in London and dance with somebody else, on the biggest entertainment show on television, with so much attention around her. But Ben has never held me back or told me I can't do it, and he completely trusts me.

The fact is that *Strictly* gave us so many amazing opportunities and experiences that we were both really grateful. It gave us the financial stability to open the studio and buy a house; it opened up the world of theatre to us so that we could do our own tour together. Then there were the other shows and events we were asked to dance in across the UK – it gave us a platform. And that first series was brilliant, because Brian was such a joker that my belly was constantly hurting from laughing. He was a calming influence as well, and I liked the fact that he'd want a tea break every hour on the hour when we were in the studio. It was great for me, because I love my cups of tea.

Brian was quite a bit older than me, but that wasn't important because I was already used to teaching people of all ages, from children to adults. 'Age is just a number, Brian, just a number,' I told him. The main thing was that he was fit and up for working hard, even if he did tend to leave it until the last minute.

Over the weeks to come, we built a great friendship based on mutual respect and laughter, and our dance partnership worked well. Don't get me wrong, we were bottom of the leader board to begin with. But it was fine because it was Week One and no one left that week, so there was no pressure. It just gave us a little push going into Week Two, when we did so much better, and I still absolutely loved it. The *Strictly* family is so loving, friendly and kind that we didn't feel any stress and giggled about it instead. We went on to dance some wonderful routines and made it all the way to

Week Five, which was great. And Brian always jokes he can't have done badly because the super-athletic Aston Merrygold went out just two weeks after he did (even though Aston and his partner, Janette Manrara, were a shock exit, to be honest).

Most importantly for me, Brian and I became solid family friends forever. He and his wife, Anne-Marie, took me and Ben under their wing; they welcomed us into their home and family. Brian treated me like a daughter, probably because I was the same age as one of his girls. He loved Ben and used to say to him, 'Come on, Ben, propose to Amy. Get a ring on it.' We'd go around every weekend on a Sunday night and have a takeaway and watch the show together with the family. We're still good friends to this day.

I've always thought that winning *Strictly* would be amazing, but my job is less about winning and more about making the celebrities fall in love with dancing. I'm lucky enough that I get to do *Strictly* again, but this is their one and only opportunity and you just want to give them the best memories and the best fun. The time of their life. It's a wonderful experience and a rollercoaster ride. At the end of it, you've made a friend for life.

On *Strictly*, you want your celebrity to be the best they can be. You can't really compare yourself to the other competitors, because you're all doing different dances every week – everyone's on their own journey. Some have a little dance experience; others haven't. There are people with disabilities; others are dancing in same-sex partnerships; you can only really focus on yourself. Getting caught up in the competition stops you focusing on getting better, so I always say to my celebrity, 'Your only competition is yourself.'

In the first series I did, my time dancing on *Strictly* was far from over when I was eliminated in Week Five. I literally finished that weekend with Brian – we got voted out on the Sunday – and on the Monday, I started practising a jive with a new partner. They used to do a *Strictly* special as part of the fundraising BBC TV telethon *Children In Need*, and this time it was the battle of the *Blue Peter* presenters. I was part-nered with Mark Curry, who was a *Blue Peter* presenter when I was born, and Mark and I went on to win the *Children In Need* competition. So I'm proud to say that I've got a *Strictly* trophy at home!

After that, I went straight into practising for the *Strictly* Christmas special, dancing with the wonderful Colin Jackson, almost ten years to the day since he'd followed Gino's and my journey to winning the Welsh Open Championships with BBC Wales. Colin and I did a rumba and got four nines, which was a great result. We're still good friends and he came to my wedding.

So that first year of *Strictly* was amazing, as I was able to experience a bit of everything: the main show with Brian, all the fantastic group numbers, *Children in Need* and the Christmas special. And during the Christmas special we got to perform the opening group number at Buckingham Palace for Camilla. Those five months of my life were just so cool and unbelievable. There were many moments when I had to pinch myself to be sure it was real.

Just imagine if I had run away scared on that first day of rehearsals! If Ben had come down from the Midlands to pick me up and take me home? Think of all the wonderful times I'd have missed. It was a valuable lesson for me.

Whatever happens, and however scared you are, try to be brave and face your fears. Don't listen to the voice that tells you that you don't deserve to live out your dreams, or that you're not worthy of your achievements or success, because you are. If you stand strong and show guts in the face of your worst nightmare, your courage will pay off, because it will give you strength to face future challenges.

Whatever the outcome, just knowing you can push through fear and insecurity will make you stronger.

At least, that's what it did for me.

Could the year have ended any better? I got home from *Strictly* just as the finishing touches were being made to our new dance studio. Ben and I were putting on a New Year's Eve party to celebrate the opening. Our families were coming and some of our closest friends. I'm not from the Midlands, so it's only really through the dance school that I can make friends locally and our 'dance family' were all invited as well.

Over the course of the evening, Ben and I were going to put on a New Year's Eve showcase, before the big celebrations started. While we were practising, Ben said, 'I want you to walk off at the end of the rumba, OK?'

'What?' I said. 'That's rubbish. I want to finish with big lifts and tricks. I've just been on *Strictly*. I want to show off!'

We had a big argument about it, but Ben wouldn't give in. For the rest of the day, he kept saying, 'Please, at the end of the rumba, just walk off.'

I was so busy organising table settings and preparing all the party bits and pieces that eventually I said, 'Yes, whatever!'

But when the showcase started, I noticed that Ben was shaking. *What's he got to be nervous about?* I wondered. *He's danced in Blackpool this year so why would he be worried about performing in front of friends and family?*

When the rumba finished, I walked off, as Ben had asked me to. Actually, I stormed off, annoyed that we hadn't ended with a flourish. But as I left the dance floor, the whole room erupted into screaming. *What's going on?* I thought.

I turned round to see Ben on one knee and holding up a ring. He'd had it hidden in his shoe! The noise got louder, the kids were jumping up and down. My parents were looking at each other, as if to say, 'Is this part of the show or is it for real?'

Time stood still as it dawned on me what a beautiful, unforgettable moment was unfolding before my eyes. Ben was proposing to me in our very own dance school, the school we'd always dreamed of setting up. We were surrounded by the people we loved and cared about, who had helped us fulfil our dreams. We'd tested what it was like to spend time apart and whether it worked for us. And we'd got through it.

So of course I was going to say yes.

Chapter 8

Showing your vulnerability lets others know they are not alone

I tried to play down my gut problems for years. I thought if I told people about it they would see me as weak. And I didn't want to be known as 'Amy with Crohn's disease'. So although there was no hiding it when I collapsed in agony with tummy pains, in my day-to-day life I tried to conceal my Crohn's. It's not going to define me, I insisted. It's not getting in my way. I'm 'Amy the dancer'.

After a flare-up, I used to push myself and go back to dancing way too soon. It took years and years for me to learn my lesson. Even after I joined *Strictly*, I didn't have a stop button. Ben used to have to take me aside and say, 'OK, you're going to have to calm down a bit. Just relax for a second. Take a deep breath. Do you need to have a day off?'

'I'm fine,' I'd say.

I didn't want to go slow. Or have a day off. I just want to be active all the time.

A lot of people seem to think that something like Crohn's only affects you when you're having a flare-up. They don't realise how much it affects you in the day-to-day. Crohn's causes ulcers and inflammation that narrow the intestine, making it painful to digest food, so it's in the back of your mind every time you sit down to eat.

I can have anything that's easy to digest, but if the gut has to work really hard I just can't eat it, because of the pain it causes. Think about how hard it is to chew a steak or a pork chop, or even just a burger; then think about my bowel, with all the inflammation and ulceration, trying to break down that steak, chop or burger in the digestive process. You're making the muscles work so hard that the ulcers weep and the inflammation becomes hot and sore. Sometimes my stomach says, 'Nope, we're not doing this', and then I'm sick.

After my first Crohn's attack at the age of eleven, Mum started writing a food diary of what I was eating. She noticed that I was poorly every time I had red meat or tomatoes, so I've not eaten either since then. As I got older, and especially around the ages of eighteen and nineteen, when I was really ill, I went on an elimination diet to rule out the things that could cause a flare-up. I had to be really disciplined about it: I went gluten-free for a few weeks, I cut out dairy for a while, and Mum recorded how I reacted.

That's when we noticed a link with food that had a skin on – and there's lots of foods with skin on, from cucumbers and red peppers to peas and sweetcorn. I don't eat anything with skin on now. If I go out to a restaurant and order a salad, all I can really have is lettuce and avocado, unless I ask the chef to peel everything. It's different at home because I can take off the skins, which allows me to eat a lot more. Never tomatoes, though, which have seeds as well as skin and are too hard for me to digest. I don't eat nuts or bread, either.

I take supplements like vitamin C, because my bowels don't

absorb all the nutrients I need, and I give myself a phosphate enema once a day because they don't open on their own. I also take daily medication, and that comes with side effects. Steroids are one of the best drugs for calming down inflammation, but although they make me feel better, they create water retention, making my hips, thighs and bottom bloat and my face puffy.

✦

When I was younger, I couldn't help feeling self-conscious when my weight fluctuated. A thoughtless comment could cut me to the core. When I've been really poorly, the pounds have dropped off me and I remember another dancer coming up to me at a competition and saying, 'You need to eat a Big Mac, you do.'

She said this without realising the hurt she was causing, or what I was going through. I wasn't trying to be skinny, I had no option, I was unwell.

I went on a course of steroids that bloated me out and a few months later, another competitor shouted out, 'Fat ass!' as I was walking onto the dance floor. 'Thick middle!' her mum shouted next.

They probably had no idea of how it would affect me, but I felt humiliated and embarrassed, and their remarks will stay with me for the rest of my life. I was only twenty-one then and still trying to deal with my condition, yet even now, more than a decade later, every time I go on steroids it's the first thing I think of – and I go on them a few times a year.

Years later, I worked with a sports psychologist who compared the impact of a hurtful remark to knocking a nail into a piece of wood. When you take the nail out, there's still a mark left in that piece of wood, and it's the same with your self-esteem.

At the time, I just had to get over it and carry on. I wanted to be judged on my own merits and told myself that putting on a few pounds – or losing them – doesn't take away from your talent as a dancer. And if I hadn't come here today to compete, I'd think, my Crohn's would be winning – and that's not happening.

Today, I try not to take it to heart when I'm photographed in an unflattering light and people make spiteful comments about my size on social media. But sometimes it can upset me, as I always want to look my best on the dance floor. The thing is, you never know why somebody is a certain size or shape. When I'm slim, it's not because I'm trying to watch my weight – I've been poorly. And when I'm bigger, I haven't been sitting there eating chocolate bars for the last six weeks – it's my body reacting to a high dose of steroids or, in more recent times, chemotherapy.

✦

I am mostly able to control my Crohn's with drugs and diet. But even if you're in remission (when you're not experiencing symptoms), having a chronic disease is seen as a risk factor by some employers and backers. It's happened to me loads over the years, so when I was offered the job on *Strictly Come Dancing*, my parents said, 'Don't get too excited until they know about your Crohn's disease.'

In an ideal world, I wouldn't have worried about it, because that'd have been a case of discrimination, wouldn't it? But experience had taught me to be wary. I hadn't forgotten the rejections at dance tryouts that had hurt so much when I was younger, and I'd been turned down for dance events and shows in later years for the same reason – I was seen as a risk because I had Crohn's disease. It was frustrating: I wanted to progress as a dancer and sometimes didn't know which pathway to take, because I kept getting knocked back for something that had nothing to do with my dancing. When my style or technique needed work, I could do something about it, but there wasn't much I could do about my health condition.

It always felt unfair, because Crohn's doesn't discriminate over who you are as a person or take away your talents, work ethic or humanity. OK, I might have time off sick because my tummy is bad, but when you know the horrific pain of Crohn's disease, nothing else touches the sides, so I'd never take time off for a cold or a headache. It balances out at work and in my dancing: because I've had Crohn's for so long, I always think I can push myself that extra bit in rehearsals (and when I do I feel proud and fulfilled). It's easy to give up when times get tough, but you don't realise how much more is in you until you try.

Strictly was the first job I'd had in the dancing industry where my Crohn's didn't seem to matter. It was such a breakthrough moment for me that, although I've mentioned it before, I still love going back over it. They just told me to include it in my insurance form and didn't for a second reconsider me. 'If you can win Blackpool, you can do *Strictly Come Dancing*,' the executive producer said.

I left that meeting with the biggest smile on my face. I felt stunned and happy as I walked through London, thinking, *Gosh, they're not worried! I've got Crohn's disease and I'm still going to be the first Welsh professional dancer on* Strictly, *the biggest dance show in the world on TV.*

It meant so much to be accepted.

Meanwhile, in the dancing world, I was told, 'Good for you. But, you know, you only got that job on *Strictly* because people feel sorry for you . . . '

The *Strictly* producers were as good as their word. Inevitably I've had times where I've been poorly over the years and, whenever I've had a flare-up, the team have put things in place to help me. They've done all they can to support me through it and I'm grateful for their help in making sure that Crohn's hasn't affected my ability to do my job. I think everybody who suffers with a chronic disease deserves that kind of support. We've not asked to have this illness and it's punishment enough having to live with it every day for the rest of our lives.

I hid my Crohn's the first year I was on the show. I wanted to prove myself as a dancer first, which was silly of me, really. I guess in the back of my mind was the fear that celebrities might say they didn't want to dance with me because of it, although I'm sure no celebrity ever would have actually said that. But because of what had happened to me in the past, that thought was always there.

I didn't mention it to the other professional *Strictly* dancers in the beginning, either. It was my first time on *Strictly* and I didn't want it to get in the way. I wanted them to get to know me as me, first. Of course, Neil and Katya already knew about

it when I joined the show, because we were friends. We both
had the same coach in Richard Porter and often went out
together in LA while we were training with him. And after
I moved in with Oti, it was inevitable she would find out at
some point. As it happened, Oti went into the bathroom to
get some toothpaste one day, opened my cupboard, saw a
stack of medication, and said, 'What's all this, Amy?'

When I sat her down and told her about my Crohn's, she
had a little cry. It really touched me; she's a lovely, caring
friend. Actually, it was a good job that she found out when
she did, because I had a flare-up a couple of weeks later and
she was up all night looking after me while I was being sick,
and in the morning, she rang the producers for me to say,
'Amy can't come in today.'

I couldn't take time off *Strictly* rehearsals without explain-
ing why, obviously. Still, I didn't go into masses of detail with
my fellow pros, or go out of my way to tell them absolutely
everything, as I had with Oti. If I'm honest, I was worried
what they would think.

They were absolutely great when I did finally tell them
all about it, and since then they've seen me collapse and be
taken off in an ambulance quite a few times. They've all been
really lovely: Katya has come with me to hospital and sat with
me until the early hours of the morning; Oti has joined me
there late into the night, after a long day filming. Dianne is
always checking in on me when she knows I'm not feeling
well, and if the boys are in any doubt they'll say, 'Nobody's
lifting Amy today.'

There have been some funny situations along the way.
While I was dancing with one of my celebrity partners,

Karim Zeroual, for *Strictly*'s Halloween Week, Ben was hosting a Halloween party at our dance studio for all the kids and the other dance teachers. *Strictly* was on the TV and Ben turned it up loud to watch me dancing with Karim, but as soon as I came out to walk down the stairs, he could tell from my face that I wasn't well. Karim and I didn't have particularly great scores after we danced, and Ben was worried that I'd find myself in the dance-offs. This is going to kick off her Crohn's, he thought.

Without waiting to see if we were in the dance-offs (we weren't) and still dressed as a skeleton in his Halloween outfit, he left the party, got in the car and drove to London. He was waiting for me when I came out of the show. 'What are you doing here?' I asked, bursting into laughter. 'And what are you wearing?'

'You know why I've come,' he said. 'You weren't looking well. There was no doubt about it, so I drove down to make sure you're OK.'

I felt better when he took me home after the show and made me rest properly, and I think he felt reassured by being with me. I wasn't great during the week to come – I was training up in Manchester with Karim – and Ben came up and stayed with me each night after he'd finished teaching, so that I wasn't on my own, just in case I was poorly.

There have been other instances when I've been unwell and *Strictly* have rung him to say, 'Amy's going off in an ambulance.' He always drops whatever he's doing and within a couple of hours, or as soon as he can, he's with me. If that's not possible, he looks out for me from afar. So when I had a flare-up in my hotel room while I was on a dancing tour,

Katya rang him immediately. Soon she had Ben on my phone and the ambulance on her phone, and she was trying to explain what was happening to me into both phones at once. Ben stays so calm in these situations. He knows how it's going to go – he's so used to it – so he tried not to get alarmed when he heard Katya shouting, 'Bring a defibrillator!'

'No, Katya, that's not what she needs . . .' he said gently.

In the end Katya gave up trying to mediate the call and put the phones together so the paramedics and Ben could speak directly to each other.

✦

There was a sense of freedom in being able to open up to my *Strictly* family. It was great to think I'd stopped hiding and could be true to myself. During my second series, the producers and dancers started saying, 'Why don't you speak out about this and what you go through?'

Deep down I'd always wanted to speak about it openly, because I wanted to help others, but I hadn't the confidence to do it. Now, I realised that it was quite selfish of me to want to hide away.

Just after the series came to an end, I came home and read a beautiful letter from a little girl who had heard about my Crohn's through a family friend. It affected me so much that I can remember the letter by heart:

Dear Amy,

    My name is Lacey Ann. I'm eight years old and I've just been diagnosed with the Crohn's disease and after researching the Crohn's disease I think it's amazing that you've got your own dance school and you're on *Strictly Come Dancing* and it made me realise that I can achieve my enormous dream of becoming a vet. It would be the best thing ever to meet you.

Lacey Ann, Year 4

Oh my goodness, I thought. *Knowing that a TV dancer has 'the Crohn's' has had a really positive impact on her.*

We met up straight away, and I started thinking about what it would have meant to me to have a role model to look up to when I was a kid. Crohn's disease wasn't spoken about on TV or in magazines back then. None of my friends knew what it was, so it was so hard for me to explain what I was going through. If I came out in public about it, I realised, then Lacey Ann could turn to her friends and say, 'You know what Amy's got? That's what I'm suffering with. We have matching teddy bears that we cuddle when we're in pain.' (True!)

Here I was, in a position to pass on a message of hope and encouragement. How could I turn this chance down? I could let my fellow sufferers know that there is light at the end of the tunnel. Tell people about the importance of pushing for a diagnosis and the correct treatment. And say, 'Look what I've managed to do, despite having Crohn's!'

And then there was the bigger picture – the chance to raise awareness of the challenges and suffering around Crohn's and colitis; to spread understanding of the impact on the families and loved ones of people with chronic diseases; and, more generally, to call for a more compassionate attitude to illness and disability in society.

I joined up with Crohn's & Colitis UK, a charity that offers support and services to people with chronic gut problems, including a helpline. I helped them with a campaign called 'It Takes Guts to Talk', which was about encouraging people to be open about their symptoms. It's terrible to think of people suffering in silence, because they're ashamed to talk about what's happening to their bodies. We wanted to reduce the stigma around discussing poo, bowels and bottoms, so that anyone affected by gut problems would feel less embarrassed about bringing up the subject with their GP, relatives and friends. We were trying to drive home the importance of taking that first step towards diagnosis, because no one can see it until you say it.

In the past, I'd read articles about Crohn's that glossed over the reality of what you go through. *Now*, I thought, *I can speak for those who suffer like me*. It changed everything. Suddenly I was on a mission.

I did an interview with *Hello!* magazine to highlight the 'It Takes Guts' campaign. It was the first time I talked about my Crohn's disease publicly and it was pretty scary. Was I doing the right thing?

I had a lot of sleepless nights worrying that it would harm my career. But the response to the campaign was so positive that I had to stop fretting. The Crohn's & Colitis UK helpline was flooded with callers and that led to an increase in the number of people going to their GP to talk about gut problems. It was a fantastic result.

Towards the end of my third series of *Strictly*, BBC Wales approached me with a proposal for a documentary about living with Crohn's. I hesitated again. Making a documentary is a much bigger step than doing a magazine article. But then I thought about how Crohn's always seemed to be misrepresented on TV, and how I, as a viewer, was always thinking, *It's not like that!*

The response to the campaign with Crohn's & Colitis UK had shown me what a difference it could make when someone from the telly stood up and talked about something like this. Now BBC Wales were giving me the chance to reveal the stark reality of living with Crohn's. Warts and all, no holds barred, the full toilet.

'It could be so helpful for people,' Laura Martin-Robinson, the director, said.

As I'd already spoken about it, I thought, *What have I got to lose by taking it further?*

✦

It was scary to show myself at my most vulnerable, but making *Strictly Amy: Crohn's and Me* turned out to be an empowering experience, all told. I met some incredible people who also suffer with Crohn's and colitis and learned a lot more about my condition, too. There were some really painful moments, though. It was difficult sitting down with my parents to recall the dark times we'd been through before I was diagnosed. But one of our aims when we started filming was to show the impact of illness on loved ones as well as sufferers. We knew how important it was.

My mum talked about how difficult it was living with the unpredictability of my illness. 'You'd think, well, this has been a good week. This has been two good weeks. We've had six months ... Suddenly, unaware, it happened again,' she said. 'It's the hardest thing in the world seeing your child in agony, without energy, and not being able to do anything.'

My dad was close to tears as he remembered one really awful Saturday morning when I was set to go to a big competition, but instead ended up in a hospital bed with two intravenous drips in my arms – and then one of the entry points became infected. Poor Dad, he was struggling to get the words out, he was so upset.

'You were so ill,' my mum said. 'We could see it. Why couldn't everybody else? Why couldn't the [health] professionals see how ill you were? And that's what was so frustrating.'

If my parents were willing to reveal their vulnerable side to the cameras, I wanted to show the reality of Crohn's from my point of view, as well. So I allowed Laura and the crew to film me during a flare-up in February 2020, less than two months after my third (and the seventeenth) *Strictly* season had ended in December 2019.

I'd had a really exciting season with my celebrity partner, Karim, and we'd made it to the final of the show – my first time. I'll never forget when they announced at the start of the show, 'Live from the BBC, this is the *Strictly Come Dancing* grand final!'

Hair and make-up had just made their finishing touches to me and Karim, and we looked immaculate. We were waiting for our cue, trying not to explode with excitement, and then we just couldn't help ourselves – when we heard that announcement, we started jumping up and down and screaming at each other. Hair and make-up looked on in horror in case we messed up all their brilliant work, but they needn't have worried: when our names were announced we smoothed ourselves down and calmly walked down the stairs, looking perfect. No one would have guessed we'd been behaving like excited little kids seconds earlier.

I remember taking a moment beforehand to think, *Wow, look how far I've come! Seven years ago, I was in hospital being investigated for Crohn's and now here I am in the* Strictly *final.*

The series ended on 14 December 2019, and then in January and February 2020 me and Karim went on the *Strictly Come Dancing* live tour across the UK and Ireland. I did thirty-three shows over six weeks and that's tough on any dancer's body, and I had the added complication of my illness. So I guess it didn't come as too much of a surprise when I became poorly – I think I knew I wasn't right towards the end of the tour, but somehow I kept going, because I had to. My mind was telling my body, 'You've got to get through this. You can't let anyone down.'

The final show was at the O2 arena in London. After seven months of dancing together, we were going out with a bang, performing in front of 10,000 people. Karim and I did two dances, the quickstep and jive, and I loved every minute of it. But after the show, I collapsed.

The documentary crew filmed me being endlessly sick into a bucket in my hotel room; they came to the hospital and filmed me lying in bed looking dreadful. We couldn't have shown a starker contrast between the performing side of me – with make-up, fake tan, big time glitz and glamour, stones and costumes – and the pale, lifeless person I am when I'm poorly in hospital, with dark circles around my eyes and a look of sheer misery.

'My body takes over and I'm not Amy any more,' I told Laura. 'I'm Amy with Crohn's, and I hate that.'

They filmed the good stuff too, as I weakly scrolled through my phone and read out messages from my *Strictly* family. The first one was from Katya: 'Sending all my positive energy and love.' And then a message from Oti: 'Are you in hospital now? I'm coming. Which one? And don't tell me no.' But I think it still shocked a lot of people to see how ill I looked.

One of my main reasons for making the documentary was to do justice to fellow sufferers and give hope to people seeking a diagnosis. So when I was better, I interviewed Professor Jeremy Sanderson, one of the leading experts on Crohn's, about what we know about chronic gut illnesses – and the possibility of finding a cure in the future.

I opened the interview by saying, 'We've known about Crohn's for nearly a hundred years, and we still don't have a cure . . . '

'We just don't seem to be able to get down to that initial trigger,' Professor Sanderson agreed. 'It's clearly a very complicated process going on in the gut.'

He pulled up some pictures to show me the difference between a healthy gut and one affected by Crohn's and colitis. 'Normally, it's a bit like the inside of your mouth, relatively smooth,' he said. 'Sometimes you get mouth ulcers, sometimes it gets sore. Crohn's and colitis are like that, but big time.'

He pointed out the difference between the smooth lining of the small intestine and colon in the scan of the normal gut, and the ulcerous, thickened intestine and swollen areas in the scan of the Crohn's-affected gut. Even I was taken aback by the contrast.

'I'd be really intrigued to know exactly why I got Crohn's,' I told him.

He said that I was most likely born with a genetic predisposition to Crohn's, which we already knew was the case. 'Those genes play against what we call the environment,' he went on, adding that stress, smoking and diet were huge factors.

I'd heard that he and his team had been developing a new treatment for Crohn's disease, so of course I was very curious about that.

'Our vaccine is aimed at showing the immune system how to handle bacteria,' he explained. 'The knock-on effect of that would be for the inflammation, we would hope, to then get better.'

'And what timescale are we looking at for this vaccine?' I asked.

'I think we're talking a good two years. But two years is not a long time in Crohn's disease. We've been waiting a long time.'

That was before Covid. Of course, when Covid began to spread through the world, work on this type of vaccine was halted and every immunisation expert in the UK turned their attention to developing the Covid vaccine. Well, you can't stop a vaccine halfway through its development, so now they've got to go back to square one and start all over again. That takes years of scientific research and testing – and before they even start, they've got to get the funding to do it.

I hope it will happen soon, because anything that calms

gut inflammation will improve the lives of at least half a million people in the UK who are living with Crohn's disease or ulcerative colitis, which affects 1 in 123 people. Medicines are improving all the time, so I would like to think that in my lifetime a cure does come about. You've always got to hold on to hope, as I say. I try to be as positive as I can.

A vaccine would transform many people's lives. But, for now, the main solution offered to many is surgery, and Professor Sanderson said it was something I needed to think about.

'How long would it take me away from dancing, if I was to have surgery?' I asked him.

'There would be every chance that if everything goes swimmingly, you'd be back dancing properly six to eight weeks later.'

He could see from my expression that I didn't like the idea of taking so much time off. 'With Crohn's disease, you have to see the bigger picture,' he added gently.

But I couldn't bear the thought of not dancing for two months. Little did I know that having cancer would involve a far bigger sacrifice than that.

I was happy with the documentary when I saw the final edit, but terrified in the days leading up to it being shown on TV, if I'm honest. *How are people going to perceive it?* I thought, panicking. *Will it help them?*

Luckily, the response was incredible. Thousands of people messaged me and the BBC, saying how much they'd loved it and how grateful they were that we'd shown the reality of what it's like to have Crohn's. It turned out to be one of the most rewarding things I've ever done – from raising awareness for the Crohn's and colitis community, to the friends I met along the way.

It felt like I'd ripped off a plaster – and now I could just be Amy, at last. I didn't have to hide anything any more. I could just be open and honest about what I go through. I don't shy away from talking about my Crohn's now when I'm doing a dance show or I'm on TV, doing an interview. I tell everybody. While I didn't tell my celebrity partners before, now they can't shut me up about it.

I want to inspire dancers, artists, performers, athletes – and anybody with a chronic illness – by showing them a person with Crohn's disease who has gone on to become a British dance champion and dance on the UK's biggest TV show. I want people to know that having something like Crohn's doesn't have to define you. It doesn't have to stop you. Yes, it might take us longer to get there. But you can get there in the end. I hope also that I've helped educate employers, family members and friends of sufferers to understand a little bit more what it's like to live with Crohn's disease.

It takes years to understand your body. And I think, as I've got older and better, I'm more tuned into how to look after myself. I listen to what my body is telling me so that I'm more aware now of the warning signs before a flare-up, which I probably wouldn't have been as a little girl growing up. It definitely helps.

After making *Strictly Amy: Crohn's and Me* I gained in confidence and came closer to accepting my condition. All my life I've been worried people would see me as weak, but I've learned that I'm not weak, I'm quite strong and brave. As

I told people after I came out about it publicly, you've got to be tough to have Crohn's disease.

It felt amazing to come out into the open. It changed my way of defining myself. I stopped insisting that I was 'Amy the dancer'. But I wasn't 'Amy with Crohn's' either.

'I'm Amy the dancer with Crohn's disease,' I started saying.

Chapter 9

Check your chest! (And if in doubt, check in with your GP)

As a dancer, you'd expect me to be body conscious. To be aware of every sinew, tendon and joint. To be tuned in to the workings of my muscles and mindful of every anatomical movement. To be in touch with my body, no less. And I felt I was.

Yet until I was thirty-two, I had never checked my chest for lumps or abnormalities.

Weirdly, I don't think I realised that people my age got breast cancer. Or not often, anyway. Apart from a few unusual cases, I thought it only happened when you got older. Even weirder is the fact that I would never have known to check my chest if I hadn't been paired with McFly's Tom Fletcher on *Strictly Come Dancing* in 2021. Yes, really! If I hadn't met Tom and his wife, Giovanna Fletcher, I might not be sitting here today. So, indirectly, *Strictly* saved my life.

✦

As I'd been a McFly fan as a young girl, I was absolutely delighted to have Tom as my partner. And it only got better. The first time I met him he was in rehearsals with the other members of McFly and they gave me my own private performance of 'It's all about Amy'. I couldn't believe it.

Within five minutes of meeting Tom, I felt as if I'd known him all my life, and since then he's become like a brother to me. It's the same with his wife, Giovanna, who is a writer, actor and presenter. The pair of them opened their arms and welcomed me and Ben into their family. It's like they were sent to me.

Tom was on tour with McFly when we were partnered up, so I often found myself in a car with him after a gig, travelling for hours to his next destination. You get to know someone really quickly when you're on a long car journey. It was lucky we got on well – it would have been awful if we hadn't.

Tom started our *Strictly* journey as the bookies' favourite to win. He was also a fan favourite and seemed to really impress the judges, especially the week we danced the paso doble. He did well and we were hoping to be in with a chance of going all the way to the final. But then in Week Nine we found ourselves in the dance-off and the judges voted us off the show. Just like that, our *Strictly* dream was all over, after working so hard. It was a huge disappointment for both of us.

'You don't look right, Amy,' Tom said, when we met up in London the following Friday to go for a walk.

'Yeah, I'm not a hundred per cent,' I agreed, putting it down to the stress and upset of our shock exit.

What happened next brought me and Tom even closer, in a funny way. We set out for a walk with Sara Davies, who was also a celebrity contestant on *Strictly* that year, but all of a sudden I started being sick. 'Tom, I need to get back,' I said.

Tom was probably a bit alarmed and rang Ben to tell him

what was going on. Ben was in Blackpool with the dance school for the weekend. 'OK, well, this is going to go one way or another,' Ben said. 'She's either going to be really sick now, or she's going to have a flare-up.'

'A flare-up?'

'Let's see how the next ten or fifteen minutes go. She's got her anti-sickness medication with her, so she can take that. Encourage her to lie down.'

I started panicking when we got back to Tom's house. Obviously, I didn't want to be ill in front of my celebrity partner and his family – in their home. You want your own bed and bathroom when you feel poorly, don't you? But there was no way Tom was letting me go home.

'OK, then can I go for a lie-down?' I asked.

'Yes, of course.'

The pain started to escalate and as I rolled around and sweated on Tom's bed, being sick, Tom rang Ben again. I think he was feeling pretty scared by this point.

'OK, she's gonna have a flare-up,' Ben said. 'Probably in the next half an hour, she's going to be screaming in pain, and she's most likely going to pass out.'

Tom was really worried. 'What do you mean, she's going to pass out? Are you coming? How long will it take you to get here?'

'Four or five hours, minimum,' Ben said. 'It's Friday, so probably longer. As soon as she starts screaming, call an ambulance.'

I did start screaming and passed out several times, so Tom called an ambulance and off I went to hospital, barely conscious of what was going on. I think he was shocked to see me in that state and it probably made him feel quite protective of me.

I stayed in hospital over the weekend. We were still in those bizarre Covid times when nobody could come and visit you, but Giovanna packed a bag full of stuff that I might need and Tom came and dropped it off for me. Given the circumstances, Ben decided to stay in Blackpool with the formation teams, so Tom picked me up from the hospital when I was discharged and I stayed at their house for a couple of days. Tom and Giovanna took care of me and wouldn't let me go home until I was 100 per cent feeling better.

Giovanna, or 'Gi', had become a good friend by then, too. Gi is the proud patron of CoppaFeel, a breast cancer awareness charity that encourages young women to 'cop a feel' and check their chest regularly. CoppaFeel organises sponsored walks in the UK and abroad to raise money for their awareness campaigns and, since I love walking, I was totally up for it when she asked me to go on a trek with her. Knowing how important this cause was to her, I wanted to help out in any way I could.

We went to Pembrokeshire in June 2022 and I found myself guiding a group of people through the breathtaking Welsh countryside. CoppaFeel's campaigns focus on promoting early detection of breast cancer in younger women, but there were ladies of all ages on the trek. Some were in their late twenties, telling me that they'd just got over breast cancer and were walking for themselves. Others were walking for somebody they'd lost, someone young. 'How old was she?' I asked one lady, when she told me about the loved one she had lost. When the answer came, I thought, *Gosh, that's around my age, and I don't even check!*

I remember going to my tent on the last night and saying to myself, 'Amy, you're trekking to raise awareness to encourage people to check their breasts and you don't even check yourself. That's ridiculous. What a hypocrite!' I think it's partly because my mum was fifty when she went through breast cancer, after it was picked up on her first mammogram. So in the back of my mind, I'd thought, *I'm fine – it's not until my fifties that I have to worry.*

But after the trek, after hearing these stories and learning the importance of checking your chest when you're younger, I started to get to know my boobs. I began checking in the June and in the following April I found the lump, so thank goodness I did start checking.

Everything changes when you find a lump in your chest. At least, it did for me. It's understandable that some people hesitate over getting their lump checked out by a doctor, because they feel scared and they'd rather not know. But I was absolutely desperate to find out whether or not my lump was cancerous. I had to wait to see the doctor because of all the plans I'd made and felt I couldn't break – partly as they were all one-off events, from my honeymoon and my brother's wedding to presenting a segment for the King's coronation coverage – but I knew from my experience of having Crohn's that getting a diagnosis leads to targeted treatment and a quicker recovery. If I had breast cancer, I didn't want to hang around feeling scared. I wanted to get rid of it as soon as I could.

When I got back from my honeymoon with Ben and my GP in Wales gave me an emergency referral to a breast clinic, the first person I rang was Rebecca, my twin sister and best friend in the world. I was in a real state and just hearing her voice made me feel less flustered. That's a twin thing, a special connection that's hard to explain, but it was also because Rebecca is a midwife and her medical training means she's brilliant in situations like this. If she was worried, she didn't show it. Instead, she focused on trying to calm me down. 'Oh, my friend's just had this and it was benign,' she said. 'Where are you? I'll come to you.'

'You can't!' I said. 'I'm filming this afternoon and doing a show in Exeter tonight.'

I drove myself to work, all of a daze, still suffering from the persistent cough that had come on a few days earlier at my brother Lloyd's wedding. The film crew could see that something was upsetting me, but what could I say? We were working on the BBC TV programme *Dare to Dance*, where I surprise people and we give them their own *Strictly* experience by teaching them to dance for an occasion that means a lot to them. This particular afternoon, I was doing an interview with a lovely lady of thirty-six, who had stage four cancer, and her husband. I did my best to put my worries aside while we were filming.

Two days later, I was still waiting for my breast clinic appointment to come through. I'd been worrying non-stop and now I began to feel frantic. My lovely friend Karla came over and instantly noticed something was up. Karla is one of our dance family mums; her daughter is a student at our dance school and we're really close.

'Everything OK?' she asked.

I smiled and tried to appear normal. 'Yes, fine!'

We talked over a few last-minute details of a formation competition the kids were doing the following day in Stoke. Then I had to rush away for a meeting. But as I was about to drive off, Karla called me back. 'You're so pale. What's the matter?' she asked, getting into the car beside me. 'Has something gone wrong at *Strictly*?'

I couldn't find the words to tell her, so I took her hand and guided it to the lump.

She frowned. 'OK ... you're thinking it's cancer? But it might be a cyst.'

I looked her straight in the eye. 'I've been to the GP and they've made an emergency referral.'

'That still doesn't mean you've got cancer,' she said. 'Let's just wait and see.'

I bent my head to hide my tears. 'I can't wait any longer! I can't sleep at night,' I told her. 'I've been looking online for a private appointment, but all the clinics are booked up.'

Like the true friend she is, kind, sweet Karla spent the next hour ringing around to find me a private appointment. 'I've found somewhere that can see you today,' she messaged me during my meeting. 'Just send me a thumbs up and I'll make the payment for you.'

I didn't even ask her how much it was going to cost. It didn't matter, I just wanted to know: is it cancer? Yes or no?

I sent her a thumbs up.

'Do you want me to come with you?' she asked.

She's a talented hairdresser and was supposed to be doing the kids' hair at the dance school in preparation for the competition the next day. 'No, you'd better go to the studio,' I said. 'We can't let them down. I'll come along later. I'm sure it's going to be fine.'

'OK, ring me if you need me and keep me posted, please.'

I drove to the clinic, where I was met by a breast nurse called Elaine, who took me in to see a consultant breast surgeon. He was very confident, very smiley. 'I'm probably going to feel this lump now and it's going to be nothing,' he said. 'I'm going to send you up for an ultrasound. They're going to explain it's a cyst and you'll be on your way and you won't see me again. If you see me – and it's not going to happen – you know we've found something.'

But when he looked at my breast and had a feel of the lump, his manner changed. I think he realised, um, actually . . .

He walked me up to the ultrasound instead of sending me there by myself, and introduced me to the radiologist, who found the two lumps on the scan and measured them on-screen. I'd Googled what breast cancer looks like, so I knew what I was seeing. The radiologist left the room and I waited anxiously to find out what would happen next.

In walked the breast nurse. In walked the radiologist. And in walked the consultant breast surgeon. I knew then, because I wasn't supposed to see him again, was I?

'We have found something and it does look like a tumour,' he said gently, 'but because of your age it could be benign. However, it's definitely not a cyst.'

'OK,' I said.

I phoned Karla. 'It's definitely not a cyst.'

'Right, I'm leaving and coming to you now.'

'Don't! You're already at the studio.' I was conscious that

it's a mammoth task getting all the kids into make-up and hair. They were all coming straight from school and we had to stick to our timetable if we were going to get everything done in time. 'I don't want anyone to suspect anything,' I added, thinking of Ben especially.

At the clinic, they explained that they were going to do a mammogram, or breast X-ray, and then take some samples of the lump, known as biopsies, which would be sent off for testing.

During the mammogram, as she looked at the X-rays of my breasts, the nurse said to me, 'I think you need to get somebody here.'

Karla phoned again. 'Are you sure you don't want me to come?'

The nurse took the phone from me and said, 'Yes, she needs somebody here.'

'OK, I'll be there soon,' Karla said.

She told me later that she'd burst into tears the moment she put the phone down. Then she thought, *No, it shouldn't be me going; it should be Ben going.*

Ben was teaching in a school in Birmingham with our other teacher, Katie. Karla managed to get hold of him after several attempts and said, 'You need to get to this hospital now for Amy. She's found a lump in her breast.'

Ben didn't question the fact that Karla knew and he didn't. He never expressed being cross about it, or the fact I hadn't told him on our honeymoon that I'd found a lump. He would have known that I didn't want him to have sleepless nights and stress on our holiday in paradise, and anyway, Ben's wise like that – he would have thought, *How's that going to help anything?* Maybe he would have been cross if I'd left it any longer, but I'd come home and started dealing with it.

I think at first when Karla rang him he thought, *It's gonna be fine. Let's not overreact. Keep calm.* He rang me, saying, 'Amy, I'm on my way, don't worry. It's going to take me about an hour because of traffic, but I'm on my way.'

In the time it took him to arrive, I had my biopsies. Afterwards, they kept me in a room with a breast nurse, who explained that if I'd been over the age of fifty, they'd probably be telling me yes, I'd got cancer. But because of my age, they were going to give me the benefit of the doubt and wait for the biopsies to come in, which would take up to two weeks.

As I left the unit carrying a pile of leaflets, I rang Rebecca and told her what had happened. 'Should we tell Mum and Dad?' I asked. They were going on holiday the next day and I knew they wouldn't go if I told them. 'It could still be nothing.'

'Keep it quiet,' she advised. 'There's nothing they can do until you get the results.'

✦

In the days that followed, the breast nurse rang me every day. She said I was going to be very sore because of all the biopsies I'd had. Also, that it did look quite likely that I had cancer, but we wouldn't know for sure until the results came through.

I was steeling myself for bad news, but Ben was very upbeat. 'It won't be,' he said. 'We're going to be positive about it.'

We were at the competition in Stoke all weekend. I didn't have a moment off, but I was very conscious of my sore breast. Early the following week, I worked on *Dare to Dance* and on

the Wednesday I had to go back to the hospital for a chest
X-ray because they were worried about my cough. I'd tried
antibiotics, antihistamines and they'd even put me on steroids, but it still wasn't shifting.

On the Thursday, we had some dance lessons booked in
London with Richard Porter, our amazing dance coach, who
was visiting the UK. It had been a very long time since we'd
had lessons with Richard and I'd been looking forward to it
for months. As my biopsy results weren't due until the following week, according to the latest update, I felt there was
nothing stopping me from going.

Our first lesson was wonderful. We were doing the cha-cha
and we loved it. For the first time since I'd found the lump
nearly three weeks earlier, I wasn't thinking about it.

We went outside for a break in the sunshine and I noticed
I'd had several missed phone calls from the hospital. I ignored
them. Even though I wanted my results, I didn't want anything to ruin this moment.

My phone started ringing again and I would have left it to
ring out if Ben hadn't said, 'Aren't you going to answer that?'

It was Elaine, the breast nurse. 'Hi, Amy, your biopsy
results are in and the doctor would like to see you. Can you
come to the hospital? We could give you an appointment
today or tomorrow.'

My heart started racing. 'Oh no, I can't, I'm in London.'

'Could you Zoom us, then?'

I hesitated.

I don't want to know, I thought. *I want to enjoy my weekend
in London and the lessons with Richard.*

'No,' I said.

Ben was looking at me as if to say, 'Amy, what are you doing?'

I think Elaine would have left it if I'd agreed to go to the hospital at some point. But now she asked, 'Are you on your own?'

'No, I'm with Ben.'

'Are you about to drive?'

'No.'

'Can I just confirm Ben is with you?'

Ben went on the phone and said he wasn't about to drive, either. Then, as we stood on the pavement outside the studio, Elaine said, 'It is what we think it is. The consultant will explain more to you when he sees you.'

And just like that, I became one of the 55,000 women in the UK who are diagnosed with breast cancer every year.

I burst into tears. Even though I'd been half-expecting it, it was still a shock. I rang my sister and cried down the phone to her. Then I rang Karla, and then my friend Jenny, who had just come out the other side of breast cancer and did her best to reassure me.

'Shall we get the train home?' Ben asked.

I wiped away my tears with my hands. 'No, let's keep dancing,' I said, conscious that we still had this time. 'I just want to carry on dancing.'

We went back into the studio, still feeling a bit stunned. Richard took one look at us and said, 'What's up, guys?' I just came out with it and Richard's expression went from disbelief to sadness.

Ben and I danced that next lesson in absolute shock. Then denial set in about what was to come and when we got on the train home, we didn't really speak.

Halfway through the journey, my dad rang. I think he sensed something was wrong. 'What's up, love?'

I tried to sound normal. 'Nothing! It's just that I'm on the train and can't really talk.'

'On the train?'

'Yes, we're coming back after our lesson with Richard . . .'

He didn't dig any deeper into why we'd cut short our trip, thank goodness. I asked about their holiday and he said they were having a lovely time.

'Send my love to Mum,' I said. 'Speak soon.'

I was relieved that I'd managed to hide my turmoil from my dad, but when Ben's mum picked us up from the station, I couldn't hold it in any longer and fell sobbing into her arms.

✦

Rebecca was there when I got home and we had a cry together. We decided we should tell Mum and Dad, so we called them the next morning, and while Rebecca, Ben and I went to the hospital to meet with the consultant, they started for home. I asked Rebecca to come, because I knew it might be very emotional for me and Ben, and, although it would be for her too, she could put her midwife's head on, listen to and take in all the medical points and know which questions to ask. We'd been through it with Mum – and Rebecca went to Mum's appointments with her for the same reason.

As I sat in the waiting room at the hospital, I was conscious that the women around me were all quite a bit older. *I'm the only one my age*, I thought. It seemed so unfair. Only around 5 per cent of the total breast cancer cases occur in women under forty. *Why me?*

'I'm not having chemo,' I told Rebecca and Ben.

They nodded. 'Let's wait and see what they have to say.'

The consultant welcomed us into his room with a warm smile and we sat down. 'So, unfortunately, you do have breast cancer,' he said. 'Have you thought about your fertility plans?'

The question took me by surprise. I was only vaguely aware that some breast cancer treatments stop your ovaries from producing eggs. I hadn't thought about it and didn't know what to say.

Apart from that bombshell, the consultant seemed very positive. He talked about the size of the lump and told me my inflammation markers were at normal levels. He explained that there are distinct types of breast cancer which originate, develop and grow in different ways and are treated differently. In very simple terms he spelled out his diagnosis for me, which was hormone receptor-positive breast cancer, a type of breast cancer that uses hormones in the body to help it grow. In my case the hormone was oestrogen, which plays an important role in the female reproductive system.

'We know how to treat this,' he said confidently. 'We're thinking: a lumpectomy to take out the affected area, a few sessions of radiotherapy and a course of tamoxifen.'

'OK,' I said, working it all out in my head. 'How long will it take for surgery?'

A lumpectomy would be all right, I thought. It's not taking away the whole breast, so I'll recover from it quickly. I'll have radiotherapy for two weeks and then take the tablets. I'm going to be fine.

I smiled. 'I can do *Strictly* then, can't I? It begins in August.'

'Well, we want to do an MRI and we need to do more

biopsies of the other lump we found,' he said, sounding a note of caution.

We left the clinic feeling a bit better than we had when we'd arrived. We rang Mum from the car and she was relieved to hear the lump was treatable and chemo wasn't on the cards. But all I could think about was that I had breast cancer. At the age of thirty-two.

When am I going to dance again? I thought, knowing I'd have to cancel the shows I had booked in over the summer.

The next day we were doing a dance show in Wales. It was a charity night and my students were coming along. 'We're going to keep this quiet, OK?' I told my parents, who were coming to watch. 'The kids and their parents are not to find out.'

Apart from telling close family members, we agreed to keep it to ourselves in order to give us time to digest it before I made the phone call to *Strictly*.

I tried not to let the stress get to me, but I was very up and down emotionally. Just before I went onstage that night, I was sick. Then I was OK when Ben and I began to dance – my worries floated away. But when we went into our final routine, dancing the jive, I burst into tears, thinking, *Please don't let anything stop me dancing!*

That week, I had an MRI scan and more biopsies. Then everything changed again. At my next appointment, the doctor said, 'The lump has doubled in size and it's grade three out of three, so it's very aggressive. We think you need a mastectomy.'

'Let's do a mastectomy, then,' I said, even though I knew it meant removing all of the breast tissue, including the nipple.

'There are specks in the other breast that we are unsure of. Also, we may need to do chemotherapy. But let's just focus on surgery to begin with.'

It's weird how quickly your life can change. In a couple of days, I went from having a diary that was absolutely packed – from not being sure how we were going to fit everything in – to having a completely empty diary. Ben and I had been all set to get an extension built on our house, but I even had to cancel the builders.

One of my big worries was that people would find out before I could tell them myself. I was going to a lot of hospital appointments; I was being recognised every time; and when you walk out of a breast clinic sobbing or not looking particularly happy, it gives everything away, doesn't it? I knew that the Girls Aloud star Sarah Harding's breast cancer diagnosis had been leaked after somebody spotted her in the hospital and posted online.

Ten of the *Strictly* pros were on tour at the time – I hadn't been able to join them because it would have meant missing my brother's wedding and filming *Dare to Dance*. I really didn't want them to learn my news on social media or in the press. Imagine Dianne finding out and then having to go on stage that night as if everything was OK! I was worried about the students at our dance school, too. Some of them were doing their GCSEs and A levels and I didn't want them to discover that their dance teacher had cancer from seeing it on their phones as they were about to go into an exam. All these things were going through my head.

It was tough telling the *Strictly* team and my friends on the show. You don't want to upset people – and it made it feel horribly real, too. They were dancing at the London Palladium that weekend and their day off was on the Monday, so I waited until then. We cried on the phone together.

All the while, I felt very alone. You can speak to your friends and your family, but no one quite understands unless they've been through it themselves. I was lucky to be able to turn to my friend Jenny, my 'pink sister' as I now call her, because the international symbol of breast cancer awareness is a pink ribbon. But Jenny is slightly older, in her forties, and has three children, so she didn't have the fertility question hanging over her, which was the biggest weight on my shoulders at the time. It's one thing to lose a breast, but I don't want to lose the opportunity of having children.

Also, we'd been there for Jenny throughout and it had been hard to watch. We were by her side on her journey, from November 2020 when she was diagnosed, to June 2021 when she rang the bell to signal that she'd ended her treatment. I saw what chemotherapy put her through, how tough and rough it was for her, how she struggled. I went through every traumatic stage with her, from diagnosis onwards. So it was all quite raw in my mind and I was terrified of going through it myself. Still, she'd had a positive outcome and Ben and I latched on to that.

✦

I knew I was going to have to put something out to the public, because I was cancelling dance shows that people had bought tickets for. And as soon as all the kids at the dance school knew, it wasn't going to remain a secret for long. People had their doubts and fears about whether it was a good idea to go public, but I felt it was the right thing to do. I thought really hard about it and decided I wanted to be in control of how I did it. I wanted to show my cancer journey in as positive a light as possible and try to raise awareness in a way that would help the breast cancer charities. I went to my agent and together we came up with a plan of action.

I went on my Instagram first, with a little post saying,

> Hey all, I've got some news which isn't easy to share. I've recently been diagnosed with breast cancer but I'm determined to get back on that dance floor before you know it. ♥ Welsh love, Amy x

I held my breath. How would people respond? I mean, you never know ...

Well, it was amazing how many people reached out and offered their support! I was inundated with messages and love that day, and my followers grew by 100,000. What really helped was hearing from women who were going through the same thing I was, because I'd almost felt like I was the only person of my age in this situation. Suddenly, I was making friends online with women in their early thirties who'd had to go for fertility treatment. Some were out the other side of surgery; others were in the same position as me and had everything in front of them. It helped so much speaking to them – just knowing that I wasn't alone, knowing that they were every bit as scared as I was. And it was so helpful, too, hearing from the ones who were a bit further along on the journey, or who had been through it and were saying it wasn't as bad as all that, and their treatment had been a success.

Speaking out put me in touch with people who could help me. I discovered a really strong community online and often found myself up all night messaging girls who'd reached out to me. And a lot of them were expressing what I was feeling. 'I know it's really sad and horrible you're going through this,' one girl messaged me, 'but it has helped me knowing I'm not the only 32-year-old going through this – and having all these issues with fertility on top.' Just that one girl's response made me glad that I'd spoken out.

Only positives seemed to be coming out of going public. I started getting messages saying, 'I've found a lump and I've been scared to go to the GP, but I'm going to go now, because of you.' It was so great to read them.

I've had thousands of messages like that since, and sometimes I think that maybe I've even helped to save a life or two – just like *Strictly*, Tom and Giovanna Fletcher, and CoppaFeel probably saved mine.

Chapter 10

Don't get bitter, get better

O ne of the hardest lessons I've had to learn is how to be patient. It doesn't come naturally to me: I don't like waiting for things; I like being active and doing things. And being patient involves having a positive attitude about the time you spend waiting, doesn't it? Which is a massive challenge when you've been diagnosed with cancer.

Waiting for surgery was horrible. That's when you feel the most alone, like nothing's being done. You're waking up in the night thinking, *I've got cancer and it's still in me.*

You just want it out of you.

Those six weeks were the hardest, longest period to get through. I felt so tense. My cough was getting worse and my mum was worried they wouldn't operate, because respiratory problems can cause complications under anaesthesia. Still, the surgery went ahead.

I woke up in my hospital room connected to surgical drains that prevent fluid collecting in your body. My chest area was very bruised and sore. I couldn't look at my breast for a while – couldn't bear to. But at least my cough had gone. And when I did pluck up the courage to take a peek at my reconstructed boob, it looked good, much better than I'd expected. I was lucky that the doctors were able to put in an implant during surgery, rather than an 'expander' that would stretch the skin in preparation for a later surgery.

When I showed it to my friend Sara Davies about two weeks after surgery, she was impressed. 'That is one good-looking boob!'

I was really pleased and said, 'Other than the nipple, you wouldn't really know, would you?' I'd been told that you can have the nipple tattooed later on, but I wasn't thinking that far ahead yet.

Maybe because of my fitness levels going into surgery, I quickly bounced back from the operation and started to heal. I spent two nights in the hospital and then my drains were removed and I was free to go home. It was June and the weather was glorious; I sat out in the garden, half in the shade, getting my vitamin D and listening to the birds singing. Friends came round and we drank endless cups of tea, and when I felt well enough, I went to the dance studio and sat watching the students have their lessons.

I recovered so, so fast. I felt better by the day. I felt so good that I told myself, 'Well, that's it! Here we go – done.'

I was ringing *Strictly* to say, 'Yep, feel amazing after my mastectomy.'

I even felt well enough to work. Exactly two weeks after my surgery, I travelled to Wales, filmed all day and travelled back. We had a barbecue at the weekend with all our friends. Everyone was amazed by how well I was.

So when I went for my pathology results, I think I went in a little bit deluded. Like, *This is easy, done it.*

✦

At my previous appointments, the doctor had addressed me with a friendly 'hello!' when he saw me. But now he didn't want to make eye contact, and I felt a jolt of fear. Mum and Dad were with me. We sat down.

'It's not what we thought,' the doctor said.

My heart sank.

'We found three tumours in total, including a tumour connected to your chest that may explain the cough you had,' he went on. 'But what shocked us most was finding lobular cancer as well as the ductal breast cancer we already knew was there.'

My head swam as I tried to take in what he was saying. I knew about the ductal cancer, which is the most common type of breast cancer. It starts in the milk ducts, the tubes that carry milk from the lobules (the milk-producing glands) to the nipple. Now he was saying he had also found the second most common type of breast cancer, which starts in the lobules and spreads out into the surrounding breast tissue like tree branches.

Two types of breast cancer. In one breast. I held my breath, waiting to hear what he was going to say next.

'So now we're suspicious of the specks in the other breast,' he continued. 'The oncologist and the breast cancer team are recommending that you have a course of chemotherapy.'

I stayed silent. I hadn't even considered having chemo. I thought it was radiotherapy, tamoxifen and we were done.

'And if they want to do chemotherapy,' he pressed on, 'you've got a two-week window now for fertility treatment.'

Two weeks? I swallowed hard. It didn't sound long enough.

He explained that it's best to start chemotherapy within six weeks of surgery. Ben and I already knew that I'd be having fertility treatment if we wanted to try for a baby later, because anyone with a hormone-fed cancer is put into menopause. But I guess the window would have been bigger if I hadn't needed chemo, so we were only just in time, as ovarian stimulation and retrieving eggs takes just over two weeks, and it's often quite hard to fit in before cancer treatment. A lot of young women with cancer miss out on fertility treatment because the timing is out.

The NHS offer an amazing fertility service for people having cancer treatment. We went for a consultation at Birmingham Women's Hospital, where the doctor I saw explained that it would begin with me injecting myself with follicle stimulating hormone (FSH) to increase the number of eggs my ovaries would produce.

I was on my period and he said, 'You need to start injecting yourself today. Otherwise, we're not going to be able to do it.'

Ben and I sat there in a daze. There were so many decisions to make, because there are so many options with fertility, and it felt so rushed.

'Do you want to store eggs or embryos?' we were asked.

'Um . . . what would you advise?'

We didn't have a chance to think about it or talk it over; we had to decide then and there. We hadn't ever had my eggs tested, or Ben's sperm, and suddenly we were worrying, *What if there are issues?*

I had an internal scan. Ben gave a sperm sample. Everything seemed fine. I started on the medication immediately and injected myself daily for the next two weeks at home. There were no guarantees, our consultant warned. Often women do not respond to fertility treatment when they're having cancer treatment. But he assured us that his team would do everything they could to make it happen. I think they try especially hard for a cancer patient, as they know it might be your one and only chance.

The good news was that I responded well, and ten days later I had a procedure to retrieve my eggs. They got nine eggs, which doesn't sound like a lot, but it is for somebody having cancer treatment. Eight eggs matured and then there was a drop-off, so by the following day it was down to seven. These went to be fertilised with Ben's sperm to create embryos. You expect quite a significant drop-off after that, because not all the eggs take to fertilisation. That's why our consultant advised us to store embryos, as they give you a better chance of having a baby than unfertilised eggs. And as we were married, we knew we wanted a baby together.

The consultant advised waiting a few extra days before freezing the embryos: they contain around six to ten cells on the third day of growing, but by the fifth or sixth day they have a more complex cell structure and as many as two hundred cells. At this stage the embryos become blastocysts and are statistically proven to have a better pregnancy rate.

It was like going on a crash course in fertility. We had to take in so many facts and stats that at times it just felt too much and I broke down. I was already an emotional mess from going through cancer treatment and surgery, and I was putting a lot of hormones into my body that were making me even more emotional. It seemed kind of ironic that Ben and I had thought that Crohn's might interfere with our ability to have children, because it can cause fertility issues. It didn't occur to us that something like this would come along.

Normally, they'd expect two or three embryos from the amount of eggs they retrieved, so we were really lucky to end up with five healthy embryos at blastocyst stage. I was over the moon when the hospital rang and told me. I was working that day with Carlos from *Strictly* and when I told him, he cried out, 'I'm a godmother!'

Dianne asked me if they were girls or boys. 'What? We don't know that!' I laughed.

✦

It was a piece of good news in among the bad, but I still had so many shadows hanging over me. What was frustrating for everyone around me was that I kept pushing back against having chemo. I just couldn't come to terms with it, because to my mind, chemo would bring loss after loss. My hair. My energy. My precious time. I couldn't bear the idea that it would put me out of action for several months of my life, possibly a year. I hate feeling tired. I hate feeling bored. And after the constant interruptions to my life and plans because of my Crohn's disease, it seemed unfair that I was having to go there all over again.

'I'm not definitely going to have it,' I said.

'But look at Jenny,' Ben kept insisting. 'She's been through it and you wouldn't even know. She's a picture of health.'

My pink sister Jenny is a friend to Ben and me equally. We met her through our dance school when we taught her daughter. You know when you meet somebody and immediately feel close to them? It was instant with Jenny, and when she saw me ill with Crohn's soon afterwards and dropped everything to help me, it showed us what a caring person she is. And when I first went off to *Strictly*, she looked after Ben, bringing him meals and keeping him company, and then it switched and Ben started going round to Jenny's house most Saturdays to watch *Strictly* with her and the kids.

Now it was inspiring seeing how well Jenny had recovered. She was feeling so much better. Her hair had grown back; she had a new lease of life and was back at work full-time, teaching.

'And that'll be you!' Ben said. 'It's just a small part of your life ...'

But we both knew what Jenny had been through. How tired she'd been, how ill and sick. There's no escaping it: chemo is a rough journey. Ben knew it, especially – he helped Jenny out as much as he could during the worst of it and did the school run with her kids when it was too much for her; sometimes I was away, but we were both as hands-on as possible to make things easier.

'Look at her now, though,' Ben kept saying.

The next time I was in Wales, I popped in to see Philip and Carol Perry, my first dance teachers. I'm as close as ever to Philip and Carol – and so is Rebecca, who moved back from Australia in 2018 after three years away and still teaches a weekly class at their dance school. We go back such a long way and they've always been so kind and supportive. And to this day, Carol rings me most weeks for a chat. Philip always says that he doesn't know who can talk more, me or Carol.

It was lovely to see them both and Carol gave me a big hug. 'So what's happening next?' she asked, after I'd filled her in on our fertility treatment.

My smile disappeared. 'The doctors want me to have chemotherapy but I haven't made my mind up yet,' I said. 'I just can't face it.'

She frowned. 'But what's the point in these embryos, then, if you don't have chemo?' she asked. 'Because you won't be around to have any babies anyway, will you?'

That's Carol for you. Everybody else was treading on egg-shells around the question of having chemo, but she tells it like it is, no sugar coating. It was a bit of tough love and I needed it.

I tried to argue with her. 'But I'll have to miss *Strictly*,' I wailed.

'OK, you'll have to miss it, but you can do other seasons of *Strictly* – or you can do just this one and that's it.'

Carol made me realise I had no choice. I needed to look beyond the next couple of years at my whole life ahead. It was about seeing the bigger picture; I couldn't get caught up in my resentment that this was happening to me. Yes, it was unfair: I'd battled Crohn's for twenty years and now I had breast cancer on top of it. But I couldn't get bitter – I had to focus on getting better. On getting back to doing what I loved most.

I thought back to the six weeks I'd spent at the London hospital having my Crohn's investigated, when I'd been in tears most days, wishing I could be anywhere else. Time went by so slowly during that stay, and as well as feeling lonely and homesick, I'd been gutted to be missing dancing and competing at the Blackpool Open Championships that spring. Yet it was worth it, because I got my diagnosis. As a result, I had access to better treatment and was able to manage my Crohn's more easily going forward. For the same reason, I needed to surrender to these coming weeks of chemotherapy in order to get rid of my breast cancer, even though it would put my life on hold.

But sometimes it's easier to think positively than to put those thoughts into practice, and I ached to be with the pro dancers, who were about to go into training for the 2023 series of *Strictly*. As the day of my first treatment came closer, I became more and more anxious about what chemo was going to do to me. I was dreading it; I was so nervous that I couldn't stop crying. I didn't realise until later that I was developing an infection that was bringing me low and probably making me feel worse. I was too emotionally drained to notice feeling poorly.

Eventually, Ben called Jenny to come and talk to me, because he wasn't getting anywhere with trying to calm me down.

Jenny understood, because she'd been through it herself, but there was no way she was going to let me duck out of chemo. 'Look at me! You would never know I'd had chemo. You're going to get through this,' she told me. 'It's going to be tough, but you're strong. Look what you've been through already. Look what you've gone through with your Crohn's. Look at how you dealt with the mastectomy. And we're going to be with you every step of the way.'

I stayed the night at Jenny's house and so, the following day, it was Jenny who pushed me through that door to my first chemo session. Maybe if I'd had my mum or Ben with me, I might have been able to wangle them round by saying, 'Please, I can't do this . . .'

But Jen wouldn't have it. She just kept repeating the same things: 'Look at me. You wouldn't even know. You're younger. You're tougher. You're stronger. You're going to ace this.'

Chemotherapy drugs stop cancer cells dividing and growing. Before you start a course, you have loads of tests to work out the correct dose for you. My chemotherapy was given intravenously through an implanted port that was put under the skin of my arm before my course began, and taken out once it finished. The port was connected to a thin tube and the chemo drugs were fed through the tube.

Having Crohn's disease meant that I was used to tests and procedures, and that definitely helped me cope with all the different treatments I had over the weeks and months of my cancer journey. I'm used to hospital stays, I'm used to injections, I'm used to MRIs and constant appointments. I've had tubes up my nose and down, loads of cannulas, and I've taken anti-sickness medication up to my ears. But for somebody like Jenny, it was all a massive shock. She'd never spent a night in hospital; very rarely was she at the doctor's or poorly, and all of a sudden she's at multiple hospital appointments, having injections and a peripherally inserted central catheter (PICC) line for administering drugs intravenously. I can't imagine how much more daunting it must be for those in this situation.

Chemotherapy often has side effects and sometimes they can be quite severe. They can reduce the number of white blood cells and increase your risk of infection, or reduce the number of red blood cells and make you dizzy and breathless. They can also cause blood clots, hair loss, sickness, vomiting, tiredness, skin reactions, numbness and a sore mouth, among other things.

But I felt OK after my first chemo session. What I didn't fully understand was how watchful you have to be of any change in your vital signs, including your pulse, breathing rate, temperature and blood pressure. Even a small rise in your temperature can be a red flag after an infusion of chemo drugs. To someone healthy, a temperature spike over 37.5°C isn't a big deal; to someone with low immunity after chemo, it can mean your body doesn't have enough white blood cells to fight an infection, and that's potentially dangerous.

My parents were staying with us, keeping an eye on me; Mum said she felt less worried about me when she was with me. When I was first diagnosed with the breast cancer, both Mum and Dad rang up their work and said they needed time off. They wanted to support me through my surgery and keep me company so that Ben could carry on teaching and running the dance school, which we all felt was really important. Then, when my course of chemo went in the diary, they booked up their annual leave to make sure they were both there for me for every treatment. I don't know where I would have been without their support. I appreciated it so much.

I had my first chemo on Thursday. It lasted a couple of hours and I felt fine leaving the hospital, but two hours later

I was being sick. I was quite poorly that night, felt better on Friday afternoon, and by the Saturday afternoon I was almost back to normal. 'You seem a bit breathless, that's all,' Mum said.

We went out for a walk. They tell you to walk after chemo because exercise gets everything moving around the body. Anyway, I'm not one for sitting around. While we were out, I got a message from the *Strictly* producers who were checking in on me. I sent a video back of me walking through the countryside. Yay! I couldn't believe how good I was feeling. They were really pleased to hear it. *Maybe this course of chemo isn't going to be as bad for her as it can be for some*, Dad thought, he told me later.

That evening, feeling tired, I lay down on the settee as we were about to watch a film. 'Don't wake me if I fall asleep,' I said.

I had a little nap and felt a bit weird when I woke up. As I went to stand, my legs went from under me and I crumpled back onto the settee. It was scary – and then I started having pains in my chest and my arm. I took my temperature. It was 38°C. 'The hospital said we need to inform them if it goes above 37.5 degrees,' Mum reminded me. She rang the hospital.

'If she's having pains in her chest, you need to ring an ambulance straight away,' they said.

The ambulance arrived within minutes and they wanted to take me in. But I was worried about picking up an infection once I got to hospital. I didn't know I already had one; I just knew I was vulnerable because my immune system was low after having chemo. 'Can't I wait till the morning? I'd rather sleep here tonight,' I said.

'No, Amy, if your temperature is high, you really do have to go into hospital,' Mum said.

The paramedics kept reassuring me. 'We'll make sure you don't go into a crowded waiting room. We'll keep you isolated.'

Mum came in the ambulance with me. Ben and Dad stayed at home, promising to come later if I needed them. The paramedics were as good as their word – as it was a Saturday night, a lot of the hospitals had ambulances queuing up to go into A&E, so they took me to a hospital further away and rang ahead to make sure there was a room waiting for me.

When I arrived, I had a chest scan because I was still breathless and the doctors thought maybe I had a clot on the lung. Blood clots are one of the known side effects of chemo, but fortunately they couldn't see one. I mentioned the pain in my arm again, but they didn't follow up on it.

'We think this could be a viral infection, which would be easier to fight than a bacterial infection,' they told us.

Mum stayed for a few hours and left at about three in the morning, after the doctors had reassured her I was in safe hands. Ben came to pick her up and take her home.

In the morning, Ben rang the hospital. 'When will Amy be coming out?' he asked. 'She's got a scan this afternoon at another hospital and we can't miss it.'

'Oh no, she won't be coming out. The doctor wants to speak to you,' he was told. 'She's being treated for sepsis and a suspected clot on the lung.'

Sepsis? Alarm bells instantly started ringing. Sepsis happens when your body overreacts to an infection and causes dangerous levels of inflammation that lead to organ dysfunction. You can't catch it from anyone – it happens when your immune system turns on itself. Sadly, Mum knew this only too well because she had lost her sister to sepsis the year before.

Ben put the phone on loudspeaker so that my parents could hear. 'She's not responding to the drugs we're giving her,' the doctor added.

Mum and Dad went into meltdown and Ben went into protective mode and rang Rebecca. Knowing that Mum would be beside herself with worry, Rebecca was straight on the phone to her, reasoning with her and trying to calm her down, even though she was upset herself. 'Sepsis is usually treatable,' she said. 'It doesn't mean anything bad is going to happen to Amy.'

Rebecca reeled off the statistics of how many people get sepsis (245,000 a year) and how many pull through (197,000). What she didn't say was that 48,000 people die of it every year. Anyway, my parents were full-on panicking by then and probably didn't hear much of what she said.

Ben was calmer and drove them to the hospital. When they arrived to find I wasn't in my hospital room, their stress levels hit the ceiling, but it turned out I was having a CT scan. They found a consultant who said that I'd gone into septic shock, meaning that my blood pressure had dropped dramatically. This could lead to potential damage to my lungs, kidneys, liver and other organs, he explained. They were about to transfer me to the Critical Care unit.

When my parents and Ben finally saw me, they were devastated to see how pale and ill I was. They watched as the team from Critical Care put me on a different, stronger dose of intravenous antibiotics, desperately hoping I would respond.

'What happens if these antibiotics don't work?' my dad asked.

There was a pause. 'The organs stop working and then the body starts to shut down,' one of the doctors said.

Dad's legs turned to jelly and almost went from under him, he told me afterwards. He and Mum were terrified they were going to lose me.

I'm lucky the doctors recognised I had sepsis, which is sometimes known as 'the hidden killer' because it's difficult to diagnose. Babies, the elderly and people with a weakened immune system are more likely to get it than others and, on average, it takes between forty-eight and seventy-two hours to become life-threatening. We worked out later that I had probably picked up an infection at the dance studio just before I went for chemo.

Awareness of sepsis is spreading among the public and NHS staff, and GPs are more alert to potential sepsis cases, but it is still the cause of tens of thousands of avoidable deaths. Sepsis can be fatal if it's missed in its early stages. Once the organs start shutting down it can kill within twenty-four hours.

Symptoms in adults include a very high or low temperature, confusion, extreme shivering or muscle pain, not passing urine, breathlessness, blotchy or discoloured skin and a racing heartbeat. Even if you can't remember this checklist of symptoms, if you or somebody else feels really unwell suddenly, it's worth asking medical staff to check for sepsis.

Fortunately for me, the stronger set of antibiotics worked. The hospital team carried on observing me until gradually my stats started improving. By early evening I was awake and answering questions, although the consultant said I wasn't out of the woods yet and still had a long way to go.

When I woke up the next day, Mum and Dad were by my bed. 'Has my temperature gone down?' I asked.

I had no idea how ill I'd been. I didn't remember a thing about it. Two days later, I was pretty much back to normal again, which surprised everybody.

I rang Ben. 'You need to come and get me,' I said, 'because I want to start going for walks again.'

After nearly a week in hospital, I managed to get home the day before my birthday. But the sepsis had weakened me and the next day my temperature spiked again. 'We've got to get you straight back into hospital,' Ben said, when I rang him to tell him.

He was at the studio teaching a class, but within minutes he'd dropped everything and was outside the house, rushing me and my mum into the car. Mum was distraught, thinking, *We can't go through this again.*

I needed more intravenous antibiotics and should have stayed in for the night, but they kindly let me go home after they'd administered them. They took pity on me because they could see how much I wanted to be at home on my birthday, having a cup of tea and birthday cake! Only as long as I went back first thing for my next antibiotic drip, they said.

I spent the next day in hospital and went home again. 'No more walks for now – you need to slow down,' Ben said.

And, for once, I actually listened.

As a kid with Crohn's, I tried to ignore the warning signs

that I was about to have a flare-up. But after learning about sepsis – how scary it is and how quickly you can go down – I made an effort to be more alert to what my body was telling me. It's a very real danger, as we know only too well in our family; my aunt's passing made us realise how quickly life can go and how precious it is.

One of the doctors at the hospital told me that having Crohn's disease puts me at higher risk of sepsis, so I was more watchful in the days following my next chemo sessions. I was really unlucky, though, and had to be rushed into hospital with blood clots in my arm after my second session. It was so frustrating. Another week in hospital. What's scary is that, as they hadn't tested the arm when I was admitted with sepsis, it's possible the clots had been there all along.

The next few chemo sessions went more smoothly, although I had days when I was very poorly and struggled. But I comforted myself with the thought that at least you know you're going to get better.

I've just got to get through these couple of days of hell and then I'll feel OK again, I'd tell myself. You can't be patient when you feel that bad; you just have to endure it.

I was sharing my feelings and experiences on social media, hoping to raise awareness of the realities of chemo and my cancer journey, while encouraging people to check their chests. And at the same time I wanted other people going through it to feel less alone, to know, 'I'm here and I'm also going through it.' And of course all their support and the good wishes that flowed back to me helped me to carry on, as well.

All along, I was getting messages from my friends at

Strictly. They kept asking me to go down to the studios and hang out. As I always like to have a goal to work towards, I was pushing myself for that; my goal was to go to *Strictly* every other weekend if I could. It was just so wonderful when I did. The production team checked that everybody around me was OK – that nobody had a cold or a temperature – and I only went on my good weekends, ten days after having chemo, when my white blood cells were back to normal levels and I was less likely to pick up an infection. Being back in the *Strictly* fold with my *Strictly* family was the best medicine. I needed it for my mental health, to have something to look forward to and keep me going through chemo. It's exciting just being backstage, even when you're not performing, because you're still soaking up the joy and glitz and glamour of it all.

So have I learned to be patient? Well, I'm getting better at it. With both Crohn's and cancer, it's been about finding a way to accept the limits set by my illness right now, but not letting them restrict the future or diminish my dreams. I have come to realise that, however much it pains you, sometimes you have to take a step back to be able to take ten steps forward.

Staying positive is about shutting down fear, overcoming negativity and looking forward rather than back. Don't get bitter, get better. Focus on your recovery. Set yourself goals. And then you can get back to doing what you love.

Chapter 11

Remember: this too shall pass

Everything changes when you get a cancer diagnosis. It pulls the floor from right under you and affects your whole outlook on life. I dreaded losing my hair so much when I started chemo treatment. Your hair is your femininity, your identity – and I wanted to stay looking like Amy even if everything else about me felt different.

I knew losing my hair was possible, though, because while chemo drugs kill cancer cells, they also target other fast-growing cells like the ones inside hair follicles. I tried to prevent it by wearing a cold cap during chemo treatments. A cold cap restricts blood flow to the scalp by cooling your head, limiting the amount of chemotherapy medication that goes there. It's not nice because it's like having a freezer attached to your head for hours on end, but it works for a lot of people so I wanted to give it a go.

You put the cold cap on an hour before you start your treatment and keep it on for an hour and a half afterwards. To stay warm, I wore gloves and woolly socks and wrapped myself up in blankets. Your body gets used to it after a bit, but it gave me an excruciating headache.

Once you turn the cold cap off, it has to stay on your head

for another twenty minutes to let it defrost, otherwise it will pull your hair out as you take it off. Your hair is like ice then and it takes forever for your head to warm up, even with a woolly hat on. I used to feel frozen for the rest of the day.

'It'll be worth it if I save my hair,' I kept telling myself.

After my second chemo session, I had to spend a week in hospital to treat blood clots in my arm, which, as I've mentioned, had probably been there during the sepsis I had after my first chemo, if only somebody had checked. Blood clots are a very scary side effect of chemotherapy, because if they travel to your heart, lungs or brain you could be in serious trouble. I had to inject myself with blood thinners after that.

I was hoping things would start to go a bit smoother when I came out of hospital after the blood clots. But it wasn't to be, and the next morning I woke up and found hair on my pillow.

Please, no, I thought.

I walked into my en suite and left a trail of hair behind me. Soon there was hair on the bathroom floor and all around the sink. My mum was staying with us at the time, keeping an eye on me because I'd been so poorly. She came into the bedroom and found me in floods of tears.

'What's the matter?' she asked.

'My hair's coming out,' I sobbed.

Mum had a little cry with me, knowing what it meant to me.

Ben came in. 'It's going to be fine,' he comforted. 'It's only a bit, you might not even lose it all.'

But it got worse in the days that followed. Karla, my

wonderful hairdresser friend, was coming over and brushing it once a day, quietly getting rid of what was falling out.

'Much gone?' I'd ask.

'Nope, it's fine.'

Like my mum, Karla knew what my hair meant to me. She'd styled it for magazine shoots, dance competitions and shows; she knew how much I loved curling it and putting it up in different styles. And Karla can work miracles with a pair of tongs.

Cancer treatment affects everybody differently and you can't always tell in advance what will happen to your hair. You might get thinning, lose a bit, or go completely bald; some treatments cause hair loss all over the body. Karla suggested cutting my hair gradually so that, if it came to it, there wouldn't be a drastic change from long hair to nothing. We both cried our eyes out the first time she took a bit off. It was that sinking moment when you think, *Oh no, there it goes.*

I started shedding even more hair after my third round of chemo and when I went to *Strictly*, I think the hair and make-up team could tell that I was going to lose it all. They were very caring about it and offered to cut it quite short, which made it look thicker. When I went the next time they cut it even shorter.

Cutting it in stages was better than doing it in one go, I guess, but it was still tough. Every part of that journey was upsetting. So many nights Ben would find me upstairs, crying my eyes out. He was brilliant. He'd come and sit with me and comfort me and let me cry. Then he'd say, 'Come on, now – it's only hair.'

'It's not *only* hair.'

He always said the same thing, more or less: 'But look, you're lucky, you've got a good chance of a cure. Some people don't have that, Amy. They would love to be in your situation, if losing their hair meant saving their life.'

He was right, there are people who don't have that option and would give anything for it. It gave me a reality check and helped to console me and to think beyond my own troubles.

Sometimes I wished I could be more like Ben; he wasn't at all worried about how I looked. For him, it's not about aesthetics or the way you present yourself – he's not that type of person – and his whole focus was on getting me through cancer and out the other side. He understood, though, and when Karla couldn't come, he brushed my hair and tried to hide the loose strands from me, so I wouldn't see what I was losing.

In the beginning, you couldn't really tell. Then my parting started to get a bit wider. One day Karla was gently brushing it through and I heard her sniffling. She didn't say anything but I could tell she was in tears. She told me later that she'd seen a bald patch appearing at the back of my head. Once she'd left my house and got into her car, she sobbed her heart out about it.

We're very lucky to have such supportive friends. Ben didn't want to leave me on my own during my course of chemo, so a few friends got together and created a 'chemo club' WhatsApp group to make sure there was always somebody to come and sit with me while I was having chemo and afterwards. It meant Ben was able to work throughout my course of cancer treatment, which was important for us.

Often, I'd go downstairs after having a sleep to find one of the chemo club in our living room. I'll never forget coming across Karla and her children, aged six and twelve, sitting so quietly on the floor reading on their iPads that you wouldn't even know they were there. 'What are you doing here?' I asked in surprise.

'I came earlier, actually!' Karla said, jumping up to put the kettle on. 'Then I went to pick the kids up from school and Jenny came in for a bit. Now she's gone to pick her kids up and I've come back here.'

'I didn't know either of you had been here at all,' I laughed.

'You've slept through it, but we've been going upstairs and peeking through the door to check you're all right.'

It seemed like nothing was too much for my chemo club friends. I was lucky, because they also understood that sometimes you need someone around, but you don't necessarily want to talk; it's just lovely to have them in the room, or sitting at the other end of the sofa from you while you watch TV together.

Before the chemo club, there was the 'Wednesday club' and Karla, Jenny and I used to meet up most Wednesday evenings. In 2020, we were there for Jen through her cancer journey and organised her party at the end of her chemo treatment. So when I got diagnosed, Karla said, 'Well, we've done it before. We'll do it again.' Bless her, she would rearrange her work to help out when I was poorly and went into hospital, and she'd bring my mum to visit me, because my mum doesn't drive. She and Jenny even took it in turns to drive me down to the *Strictly* days when I first went back to the show, knowing how hard it would be for me.

Karla, Jenny and our other friends have been rocks – they've been through every emotion with us, every piece of news; we've laughed together and cried together. They've been on the edge of their seats, nervously watching their phones, waiting for results. You can see it has meant as much to them as it has to us.

But it's funny, because there are one or two people I haven't heard a peep from since my cancer diagnosis. So you learn, don't you, who your real mates are. I'm not talking about the people who have found it painful to support me because they've lost loved ones or been through it themselves. I totally understand – it must bring it all back – and if I'm honest, I'm not sure how I'm going to feel if I have to watch someone else go through it. But even so, those friends still manage to say, 'I'm here for you', and send messages to show they're thinking about me. It's the one or two who haven't got in touch at all that I'm thinking of. You can't help but wonder why.

✦

It was Karla's turn in the chemo club slot when I went to my fourth session, eight weeks into treatment. She probably wished it wasn't, though, because I started being violently sick within ten seconds of the chemo being administered! It was so bad that after three doses of anti-sickness medication, I was still vomiting, and they had to get the doctor to bring me another dose.

The nurses thought that maybe the chemo and cold cap combined was putting my body through too much to handle. 'I think you need to decide if this cold cap is worth it,' one of the nurses said.

By then, I had lost so much hair that it was beginning to look like I was going bald. My parting was getting wider and the hairless patch at the back of my head was bigger.

'It's not really working for you, anyway,' someone else said bluntly.

Jenny, having been through breast cancer and the whole hair-loss journey, including having her head shaved by Karla, had talked to me about it the night before. Even if I kept on with the cold cap, she warned, I'd probably have to shave my head anyway, because the hair loss had already gone too far. 'You have to think of the regrowth,' she said, 'because what's it going to look like when you've mostly got long hair, but with little spiky bits going on as well?'

She explained that the hair grows back like baby fluff, and shaving it stimulates the hair follicles. 'So is it worth having a cold cap tomorrow for six hours?' she asked. 'You'll prob-ably be wearing wigs anyway, so what's the point? I'm being honest because I don't want you to go through all this pain for nothing.'

And I wanted her to be honest. She's a real friend and she had cold capped as well. She was only echoing what my par-ents had been saying, anyway: 'Why are you putting yourself through it? Don't do it.'

Ben as well: 'Why are you carrying on with the cold cap? It means you have to stay at chemo for so much longer.'

I still gave it a try. That's typical of me – tell me I can't and I will. I wasn't ready to accept losing my hair.

But now my body was saying no and it was time to make a decision. I wasn't sure it was much of a choice, though. Four chemo sessions in, there was no getting around the fact that

I was spending a lot of my day in dread – dread of waking up in the morning and seeing what was on the pillow; dread of having a shower and seeing hair clogging the plughole. When I got up off the sofa, there'd be a trail of hair. Everyone was picking up hair after me. Was I really going to carry on tormenting myself with the brushing and watching it fall out?

My next treatment would involve going on a different type of chemo and having to wear that freezing cap on my head for eight hours. I couldn't face it.

'OK, I can't continue with the cold cap,' I decided.

Karla reached for the tube to disconnect it from the cooler machine but quickly pulled her hand away. 'Ow!'

It was painfully icy to the touch. I reached over and felt it for myself. 'That's not even as freezing as it is on my head!'

She tried again and disconnected it this time. As soon as you disconnect the cold cap during treatment, there's no going back. So although it was a massive relief not to have to keep enduring it, we knew that within the next ten days I would be going bald.

I looked at Karla and we started crying. We sobbed and sobbed and sobbed. And while we were crying, the words of one of the cancer nurses came back to me – the specialist nurse who had been there when I was diagnosed. 'Let it out, Amy, cry,' she'd advised. 'You're often going to need a really good cry; don't hold it in.'

I can't hide my feelings, anyway! I cry easily when I'm upset; I'm sensitive. For me it's better than holding it in – and right then it felt like I was releasing all the dread and worry about losing my hair that had been pent-up inside me. I'm lucky in being able to open up and let my feelings out around my friends and family, because I trust them enough to let myself go. Of course, there were also times when I needed to be on my own with my feelings – there still are – and then I'd come home and sit in the shower and cry. I had to be aware of other people's feelings, too. I didn't want to drag anyone else down with me.

My sister Rebecca struggled with my hair loss, so I wasn't always that open in front of her. I started to be more mindful of this after she got upset when she came with me for a wig fitting. Mostly, it was fun trying on all the different wigs in the shop together, especially the really ridiculous ones. We laughed so much. But then, just before we left, Rebecca burst into tears. Maybe trying on wigs made her think about what it would be like to be in my position, I don't know. But she literally broke down in the shop, bless her, so I tried to keep a brave face in front of her after that.

Rebecca came down to *Strictly* with me for the filming of the show's opening sequence, when all the couples do a piece for the titles. Watching them made me feel sad. I wanted to be caught up in the excitement of *Strictly*, doing what they were doing. And I was missing every aspect of dancing, but I had my port in my arm and couldn't really dance. The emotion welled up inside me and when Katya and Rebecca were helping me put my wig on, the tears started. My hair was thinning, I couldn't do what I loved the most: I didn't feel like myself and was overwhelmed by feelings of loss.

Katya and Rebecca helped me pull myself together and when I was feeling a bit better, I went off to the wardrobe department. They did a good job of encouraging and building me up again, but it must have taken its toll because when

I came back into the dressing room, I walked in on them having a cry together.

I walked straight back out again, so they didn't see me. *They're being so strong for me and I must be strong for them*, I thought.

✦

Deciding to shave my head was the hardest step, just over halfway through my treatment. It was a couple of days after I'd stopped with the cold cap and I realised it was time to take control, after months of having no control over anything.

I texted my friends' group chat – which included my chemo club friends – and said, 'That's it, I'm doing it. Tomorrow I'm shaving my hair. But I want it to be fun. I don't want it to be a sad thing. Let's all get together at Jen's house and make this as positive as we possibly can.'

I rang Karla. 'Can you bring the clippers from the salon tonight?'

Poor Karla has shared so many difficult moments with me and Jen that she says she almost feels like she's been through breast cancer herself. 'Yeah, OK,' she said now.

We gathered at Jen's because she's got a lovely big, open kitchen-diner and garden. I was glad that Mum and Dad were staying with us that weekend. Then my sister, my brother, his wife and their little boy turned up to surprise me, all the way from Wales! Surrounded by friends and loved ones, I felt braver and stronger. My mum said afterwards that she had been dreading it, but it wasn't as bad as she thought it was going to be because all the right people were there.

Don't get me wrong, it wasn't easy. But we tried to make

it as fun and uplifting as possible. Before Karla got out the clippers, we drank Nosecco, which is non-alcoholic sparkling wine, and made a video for Instagram. Of course there had to be a dance element, so we also did a TikTok dance routine; Dianne sent over some ideas for the choreography and some other *Strictly* pros chipped in on FaceTime. There were some non-dancers among us, obviously, and watching my dad have to learn the dance was definitely a highlight.

Everyone took turns to cut a lock of my hair and then Karla cut my hair short and shaved my head. I tried to keep smiling, but it was really hard – for both of us. Karla was apparently in bits afterwards, although she hid it from me, and it's no wonder she felt emotional: in the space of three years, she'd had to shave the heads of two of her closest friends because of breast cancer treatment.

The first time I looked at myself in the mirror, the shock of seeing myself bald made me laugh. I'm still getting used to it now. But although my chemo treatment is over, I can't help feeling that I'm still being punished as I wait for my hair to grow, knowing it will take years to get it back to how it was, and my reflection is a constant reminder of what I've been through. I look at people with their lovely long hair and I envy them. Yeah, I've got fantastic wigs, but it's not the same. It's not your own hair and doesn't feel natural at all.

At first, I couldn't let anyone see my bald head, even though I'd put an Instagram video out a couple of days after I'd shaved it. I did the post because I wanted to share the truth and be honest about the reality of chemo – and losing your hair is a major part of it. I think a lot of people fear losing their hair, and I was hoping it would help give courage to others who maybe were about to shave their heads or had already done so. 'I'm with you. I'm there too. Cancer doesn't discriminate,' I was saying. On a more personal level, putting it out there meant that it wouldn't be a shock when people saw me – and yet it still felt too exposing to let anybody see me in real life without a hat on, a headscarf or a wig. If the postman knocked on the door, or the builders came round, I'd straight away put a scarf on.

And then, towards the end of that week, I went down to *Strictly* again; Rebecca was coming with me and it was going to be my first live appearance on the show, a surprise appearance reading out the voting terms and conditions (the T&Cs).

I'd also been invited to the Pride of Britain awards, a celebration of extraordinary people who go above and beyond to help others, the really good, courageous people in our society. It's an inspirational event and I was among a group of *Strictly* dancers presenting an award to a remarkable man who had raised a huge amount of money for the Macmillan Cancer Support charity. Me, Rebecca and Dianne were going, together with some of the other pro dancers.

When the stylist who was helping us source our dresses asked me what I wanted to wear, I said, 'It's Breast Cancer Awareness Month, so I'd like something pink to represent that. And if it has a bow on, amazing.' The stylist sent across some photo suggestions and I chose a pink satin dress with a massive bow. Perfect!

Dianne and I did our dress fittings in my hotel room with the stylist and Rebecca. I loved the look of my dress on the hanger – it said it all – but when I tried it on it didn't look right, even though it was a snug fit. It was something to do with my big wig and the big bow – it was too much, a clash.

I had a hot flush while I was pondering what to do. I'd just been put into menopause and these waves of heat kept sweeping through me and turning me into a ball of sweat. I took my wig off to cool down and Dianne, the stylist and my sister turned to look at me. 'Oh my God!' they all said at once. 'The dress . . .'

Looking in the mirror, I could see the dress looked way better now. When I'd picked it out, I'd seen it on a model who had her hair slicked back into a bun, which is why it had looked so good. But I couldn't slick back my wig, because it would ruin it. You've got to be so careful with wigs because they're unbelievably expensive.

It was the first time Dianne had seen me face to face without my hair. 'Amy, you look amazing! You need to do this without a wig on,' she urged.

I looked at Rebecca to see what she thought. 'I hate to say this, but she's right,' my sister said.

Then the stylist chipped in. 'I didn't want to say anything, but you totally rock this and if you can't go without a wig, I don't know if this dress is right for you.'

Dianne and Rebecca kept on and on about it all night. The following day I went to film the T&Cs, wearing a headscarf. When I went into hair and make-up to have my wig fitted, the hair people said, 'We need to curl it, so don't wear the wig for the dress run. Keep the scarf on.'

Just then, I had a hot flush and took my headscarf off for a second. Dianne's eyes lit up. 'I just love this bald look,' she said. I quickly covered up again. 'Why are you putting your headscarf back on when you're feeling hot?' she asked.

I was so hot I took it off again. Just then, a couple of the pros walked past me. They didn't do a double-take. They didn't say anything or do anything.

'Just go out there and do the dress run without your head-scarf on,' Dianne urged.

I was so hot that I did exactly that. I could see the production team up in the gallery were surprised. 'She's gone out there bald!'

I did a video of the rehearsal and sent it on a group chat to Karla and Jenny. I'm not sure which of them was more taken aback, but as my hairdresser, Karla probably thought that she would be the only person ever to see my hair as it was growing back. Knowing me as she did – and I always glam myself up before I leave the house – she thought I'd never be seen without a headscarf or a wig on.

I still have the texts they sent in response:

> Jenny: I can't begin to tell you how proud of you I am for doing it without your wig. You are an inspiration. Not much makes me cry as you know, but I burst into tears.

> Karla: Oh my God, love, love, love! Can't wait for tonight.

Then Jenny texted: 'You have a platform and you've used it.' I realised she thought I'd already filmed it. Whoops!

'This is only the dress run,' I wrote hastily. 'I think I'm going to wear my wig for the real thing.'

Jenny: Oh, it has to be right for you. But
what power you have.

Karla: You're beautiful either way,
can't wait.

After the dress run, I went into hair and make-up. 'You need to do the T&Cs without a wig!' everybody was saying. 'Imagine what it would do for everyone else going through this. You've got the platform – use it!'

'I'm hiding your wig,' one of the girls joked.

I already felt a little bit exhilarated and proud of myself, just for braving it in the studio. *Should I go all the way?* I wondered. I had Jenny and Karla on at me; I had Dianne on at me, and my sister. But I was still unsure. Two days earlier, I'd been worried about the builder seeing me without my scarf – now I was thinking about revealing my bald head to an audience of millions.

I went and spoke to the production team. 'It's entirely up to you,' they said. 'We'd love you to do it without, but it's your first appearance on *Strictly* this season, so you must do what you feel happiest with.'

I felt hesitant right up until the last minute. For once, I didn't discuss it with Ben or my parents. Then something inside me said, *Yeah, let's do this for everybody else on this journey.*

I told the production team that I was going to do it without my wig. And then I went ahead and filmed the T&Cs while exposing my bald head to the world.

My phone started buzzing immediately.

The response online and on social media was just unbelievable. All the newspapers covered it and the comments were filled with love.

Then a comment on my Instagram, posted by Clara B, went viral:

> Amy Dowden choosing not to wear a
> wig on #Strictly tonight has just shown
> every little girl going through chemo
> that bald is beautiful. What a role model.

I was so thrilled to think I might be able to help to make chemo less of a burden to other people going through it, especially young girls.

'There are no words to describe the pure joy and happiness I felt last night being back with my @bbcstrictly family,' I posted in response, the following day:

> It is their love and support that gave
> me the courage to decide last minute
> to step out and brave the bald. It's
> messages like the above which is why
> I use my platform to raise awareness
> and hopefully give others confidence
> #baldisbeautful.

Now I wasn't worried about going to the Pride of Britain ceremony without my wig. In fact, I went to the awards positively showing off my bald head, hoping it would give courage to people of all ages, but especially to teenage girls who have lost their hair because of alopecia, or leukaemia or another cancer. I was seeing a lot of teenage girls going into the unit when I was in having treatment, and my heart went out to every one of them. Knowing how hard I was finding it, I couldn't imagine how awful it must be for them, so I was hoping that if their mates saw me on the TV with a bald head, they'd think, *Oh, that's like my friend at school!* It's normal. It's fine. Nothing for them to be embarrassed or ashamed about.

✦

I'm finding that I draw energy and strength from raising awareness about the things I've gone through, or am going through.

For me the most powerful message of that awards evening came from a little girl called Freya Harris, who won the Pride of Britain Child of Courage award. Aged eight, Freya was diagnosed with a rare kidney tumour and went through extensive treatment, including surgery, which must have left her exhausted. But her life turned around when her parents gave her an Australian Shepherd puppy, Echo, and she set her sights on training Echo to compete in the international dog show Crufts. That's quite an ambition for any eight-year-old! Let alone a kid who's just been through stage four cancer.

Despite loads of health setbacks, Freya's hard work and determination actually got her into Crufts. After qualifying, she almost didn't make it because she had to have a blood transfusion the night before the competition, but she got there in the end and triumphed. The judges placed her and Echo second in their category.

Freya said she did it 'to help people fight and make their dreams come true'.

Hearing Freya's story had a huge effect on me. I was sobbing away in my seat, of course! I felt inspired by her courage and joy for life.

The following day, a fifteen-year-old girl who has been a student of mine for ages messaged me:

> I meant to say last week, but forgot –
> some of my friends came out of a
> science lesson about cancer and said
> that the teacher, who is new and doesn't
> know anything about me dancing at your
> school, mentioned you and explained
> how inspiring you've been by sharing
> your journey. Thank you for being
> such an inspiration and showing us all
> that you can do anything you put your
> mind to.

Sometimes I've felt very vulnerable as I've shared my cancer journey, but getting a message like that makes it all feel worthwhile. So, if because of my platform and position I can help others in the same situation as me – or going through other challenges – I'll carry on talking publicly about my experiences of cancer for as long as people find it helpful.

Chapter 12

Don't keep your feelings in – let them go

P eople ask me if chemotherapy was as bad as I thought it was going to be. I'm not going to pretend it wasn't. But you get through it.

I already knew that it could be brutal from seeing what my pink sister Jenny went through. Anyway, there was no shortage of people among my wider circle of family and friends reminding me of all the rotten things that would happen.

'You're going to feel so tired after chemo that you won't be able to dance again this year,' I was told. 'You're going to gain loads of weight when you have hormone therapy.'

How do you know? I'd be thinking. Maybe that's been your journey, and maybe it's completely different from mine.

There was a lot of interest in my fertility, even from people I didn't know very well. 'So will you be able to carry a child? You'll have to get a surrogate now, won't you? How much is that going to cost you?'

As they fired off questions, I'd be sitting there, wide-eyed, thinking, *Do you know what? Right now, I'm fighting for my life, so that's where my energy is. Why are we going down that road already?*

'What?' I was asked. 'You're planning to go back into *Strictly* after all this?'

Seriously, would you say that to a schoolteacher or a nurse? I was thinking. *Do you want me to have a change of career, now?*

I don't believe most people want to cross boundaries and be insensitive intentionally; I think they mean well but maybe feel nervous around subjects like cancer, and either get tongue-tied or blurt things out without thinking them through first. I know it's up to me to try to gently steer the conversation to what I am comfortable with, but it's not always easy.

Before I appeared on *Strictly* without a wig, a lot of people seemed fixated on whether I would lose my hair. I think everybody knows that ultimately you're going to lose it and they're either intrigued or curious – they just want to know more. They kept bringing it up, even when I was sharing on social media how anxious I was about hair loss and struggling to come to terms with it. As a result, I think it became an even bigger problem in my mind than it already was, because I kept having to explain myself. So I was incredibly grateful for the sensitivity shown by the oncology nurses at the Sheldon Unit in Good Hope Hospital where I was having my treatment, who were positive and gently encouraging around hair loss and all the other aspects of breast cancer that you have to contend with. It's part of their training, obviously, but they helped me face up to my fears and see that there's nothing actually wrong with having a bald head.

I still found it hard to accept the loss of my eyebrows and eyelashes, though. When they fell out, it was as if the last of my femininity was going with them.

I understand it is difficult to know what to say to someone going through any type of traumatic event. If you have a friend or family member who has cancer – and I can only really speak for myself – just treat them normally. I know I wanted to be treated as normal. I understand that sometimes people don't know how to address it, but the best thing would have been to ask how I was and then take it from there. And when I was out and about and had my headscarf on, I didn't want looks of sympathy or pity. I didn't want people to feel sorry for me, but to stand strong with me.

On top of the usual chemo challenges, I went through a series of health complications that made the whole experience a lot worse. There was the infection after my first round of chemo that I've already described, when I went into septic shock and nearly died. After the second, I spent that week in hospital with blood clots in my arm. Why was that such a problem? A blood clot, or thrombus, is a collection of blood that lumps together and blocks the blood flow through a vein or artery. If it travels around your body, it's especially dangerous when it starts to interfere with your heart or lung function. I'd been told that cancer can increase your risk of blood clots, as can some of the drugs used to treat cancer, so it's important to watch out for signs like breathlessness, pain and swelling.

I was OK after my third chemo, apart from all the hair loss, but I had a mini scare after my fourth round and ended up in hospital again when my temperature spiked because of a virus and they kept me in overnight. I started dreading the days after my chemo sessions: what would happen next? But I pushed on through and told myself that one day all this would be a distant memory.

Fortunately, there were no more hospital admissions, but

from my fourth to eighth chemo sessions I suffered a lot of bone pain. Some cancer drugs cause a loss of bone density and, to counteract it, you have to give yourself bone marrow injections that help to reduce white blood cells. These gave me a lot of pain in my back and the tops of my legs, a deep ache that I just couldn't shift. The doctors prescribed strong painkillers – just in case – and recommended having baths to relax me and ease the pain. I had a lot of baths . . .

Early on, I found it hard when people brought up *Strictly Come Dancing*. I'd be at the hospital, or having chemo and not in the best of places, and they'd be straight in there: '*Strictly*! Who do you think's gonna win? Ooh, are you missing the other dancers? Who do you think would have been your celeb?'

I'd look at them helplessly, thinking, *This is not a good time. I don't want to think about who would have been my celeb, because guess what? I can't dance at all right now.*

I expected people to be more sensitive to the fact that I couldn't do what I loved. Of course, it wasn't just the pain in my bones and the port in my arm that was holding me back. Chemotherapy drained my energy and left me feeling so listless that I didn't have the urge to dance, because I wasn't 100 per cent Amy. It wasn't the same feeling as during lockdown when I felt well but there weren't many dancing opportunities. Now I just wasn't myself and it was like I couldn't get back to being myself until I started dancing again.

Being an active person, I was always going to find it a struggle to do nothing. 'It's a good excuse to read books and catch up on box sets, though, isn't it?' people said. But to be honest, I couldn't focus, because I couldn't stop my mind going into overdrive with worries and what-ifs about the future – what if my cancer comes back, what if my hair doesn't grow? What if I can't get back into shape fast enough, or fit into my dance dresses? It was torture having to sit with these sorts of thoughts on a loop while I tried to concentrate on a book or a film. Big worries and little worries circled inside my head until I thought I'd pop with tension and anxiety.

I went on social media a bit, and social media is great in many ways. You only have to look at what it's done for Crohn's and colitis and breast cancer in terms of spreading awareness and information. And it's fantastic for getting the message out about people checking themselves, especially to younger followers. For that reason, I love it, and also for the way it builds a platform for people to know each other on different levels – in my case connecting me with my pink sisters, my *Strictly* fans, my colleagues, dance students, friends, family and more. But social media is not the real world, and sometimes it's not great because there's so much trolling, filters and fakeness. There are some people who put the truth out there and that's fantastic. But so often somebody will post a gorgeous picture to show they've had a wonderful morning – the best Monday morning ever, say – when really they've done the washing, cleaned their house and dropped the kids off to school.

It's OK in moderation, but I won't go online if I'm having a Crohn's flare-up, because there I am in bed, vomiting or in agony, and then I go online and see everybody having the most wonderful time. I also gave it a miss during my bad days getting over chemo. I tried to be as truthful as I could, though, and didn't hide the reality of what I was going through; I even filmed myself having a session of chemotherapy to show what it was like. And when I had a few good days between sessions, every two weeks, I was able to share a more positive picture of my chemo journey as well.

✦

I made the most of the good days; I tried to squeeze every drop of enjoyment out of the times I was feeling well. Ben and I would have a morning out together and go for lunch somewhere; that was nice because we're usually too busy to treat ourselves in that way. Or Rebecca would come up and cook me a nutritious meal and we'd go for a nice walk with Ben. Rebecca and Ben get on really well. They have a lovely relationship, in fact.

I spent as much time as I could with my closest friends and my mum and dad – nothing strenuous, just short bursts. Sadly, I didn't get to see much of my brother, Lloyd, his wife, Holly, and my two-year-old nephew, Jacob, because Jacob was at nursery and kids carry bugs, so it was too much of a risk. It was really tough, because having a cuddle with Jacob is the best feeling. Mum and Dad could only see him on their way back from visiting me, but he was the tonic they needed after seeing me so poorly with chemo. The only time I did see him – and they made sure he was well – was when I shaved my hair. Still, I'm making up for it now, which is lovely. Jacob is the apple of everybody's eye – and obviously Lloyd and Holly think he's pretty special too! We all do.

Sometimes, on a good day, you'd find me in the dance

studio with Ben, watching a class or helping to teach. For some reason it surprises people that I still love teaching so much, especially when they see me on telly one day and coaching my students the next. I'll never forget the weekend after my first *Strictly* series ended, when I went to Blackpool with my dance school. The other dance schools couldn't believe it when they saw me getting my students ready, pinning their numbers on, giving them last-minute tips, touching up their make-up and shouting for them to do well until I was hoarse. But I'm still the same dance teacher that I was before I went on *Strictly*, and I still love the excitement of those competitions in Blackpool, even if I'm only sticking diamanté stones on dresses in the waiting room. I can't see that ever changing.

So, despite the bad times, I had some positive times over the course of my treatment. Yet the day of my final round of chemo couldn't come soon enough – my mind was always fixed on that goal. A lot of chemotherapy wards have a bell you ring to signify that you've had your last session – and I couldn't wait to ring the bell at the Sheldon Unit on 9 November 2023, the planned date of my eighth and final round. Then, I thought, my cancer journey would finally be over. Or, at least, I hoped it would. After months of anxiety and health setbacks, I was desperate to move on and start the next chapter of my life.

When the day finally came, I cried all morning. 'I'm so lucky and grateful to be able to ring that bell!' I posted on Instagram, as I arrived at the Good Hope Hospital in Birmingham with Ben. 'Will never take it for granted! Thank you to the incredible Sheldon Unit! You are all amazing NHS, all true heroes.'

My emotions were all over the place. I was in tears one minute and smiling the next, hugging the nurses and crying with my mum and dad. My family and friends had turned up to surprise me with cake, balloons and flowers, wearing bright pink T-shirts; we had a group hug and, as they wrapped me up in their love, I felt an overwhelming sense of relief that I'd finally made it to the end of my treatment.

Two other cancer survivors were finishing their chemo treatment along with me and we took photos together. 'Today all three of us rang that chemo bell! 32, 35 and 26 when diagnosed with breast cancer so, please, this is a note from us three to check your chest! Cancer doesn't discriminate,' I posted.

A lot of people on social media seemed taken aback when they saw our ages. Like me, they hadn't realised that it's not that unusual for young women to go through breast cancer. Until I went on the CoppaFeel trek in 2022, I didn't know that at my age I'm supposed to check my chest regularly. I didn't know *how* to check my breasts for abnormalities, either.

I now know that everyone's breasts are different and it doesn't take long to get a sense of what feels normal for you. The key thing is to get to know your chest and check it every month. Do your nipples, boobs and underarms look and feel the same as the last time you checked? Has anything changed?

How do you even know if something is wrong? Some people have pain, others have bleeding or discharge from the nipple; I just had a lump. If you're at all concerned, go and see your GP. The sooner you put your mind at ease, the better. And if there's a problem, it's better to catch it early, because it will be easier to treat.

Everyone's breast cancer journey is different – I can't stress that enough. Some people go through chemo before surgery and radiotherapy; others have the surgery first, like I did. There are many different types of breast cancer, including invasive and non-invasive ductal carcinoma, invasive and non-invasive lobular carcinoma, triple-negative breast cancer, inflammatory breast cancer, metastatic breast cancer and Paget's disease of the nipple. None of these terms meant anything to me before I found my lump, and I've since found out that no two breast cancers are the same. I had no clue, either, about all the drugs and treatments used to combat all the different types, or the long list of side effects to watch out for.

I didn't even know that men are also affected by breast cancer until I met a gentleman on my chemo ward who'd had both breasts removed and stitched up. He was wearing a cold cap while having a round of chemo.

'Oh, you're doing the cold cap as well!' I said. I don't know why I was surprised – I shouldn't have doubted it – as a man's hair is clearly as important as a woman's.

'Yeah, I'm hoping my hair won't fall out, because I don't want my kids to realise I've got cancer and I'm having chemo,' he explained.

As we chatted, he told me that, like me, he hadn't realised that a man could get breast cancer. It made me think I should start calling that area my chest rather than my breasts, to get people thinking about it. Now, when I'm asked, 'Why do you call it your chest?' it gives me the chance to talk about the male side of the disease. It may not seem like something to prioritise, as male breast cancer cases make up fewer than

1 per cent of all breast cancer diagnoses. But at least four hundred men are diagnosed with breast cancer every year, mostly with invasive ductal carcinomas, and people are usually surprised to hear that men can get it at all. It's important to be aware of it.

✦

In the days that followed my final chemo session, I had a lot of messages from friends and followers congratulating me. Everyone was thinking that it marked the finish line of my cancer journey. I thought so too. *That's it, done!*

Oh, if only! I must have been so focused on ringing the bell that it slipped my mind I'd be going back to the ward once a month for the next five years. How could I have forgotten that I need a monthly injection to keep my hormones at bay, so that they don't feed the cancer? It's either that or have my ovaries removed, which I didn't want.

I think we get it into our heads that when we finish chemo that's it, but you learn it really isn't.

'When will my eyelashes and everything start coming back?' I asked one of the nurses when I went back to the ward to have the port removed from my arm.

'Six weeks from your last chemo,' she said. 'It takes six weeks for the medication to completely go through the bloodstream.'

'What?' I said, in surprise. If it stayed in my system all that time, surely that meant I'd still be getting side effects for weeks to come? Yet I had spotted eyelashes on a couple of my pink sisters who had finished chemo the same week as me. 'Why is their hair is growing back faster than mine?' I asked.

'Because they're on another medication and it has different side effects, even though they have breast cancer as well.'

Of course, I thought. Because everybody's experience is different.

There was no getting around it: my journey wasn't over. Before the chemo drugs were even out of my system, I'd be having the all-important MRI scan that would show whether or not they had worked. My blood levels and other tests indicated that they had and my chest was free of cancer. But I was beginning to realise that the memory of these past few months would take time to fade – and would maybe never fade.

Perhaps it will be different when I'm feeling back to full strength, I decided, although sometimes it was hard to imagine ever feeling like the old Amy. I was alert to every twinge and ache in my body and constantly worrying that it could be a sign of the cancer returning or spreading.

I tried to focus on the positives and look forward to getting back on the dance floor. A few weeks earlier, the executive producer and series producer at *Strictly* had come up with an idea for a group number based around my cancer journey, for the semi-final show in December. It sounded so exciting – I couldn't wait to dance with my *Strictly* family again, and to tell my story through dance. It was an amazing opportunity to spread awareness of breast cancer in young women. When I got off the Zoom call with the team, I had a little cry, and then I rang Mum and Dad. 'I'm going to do a group number at *Strictly*!'

Having my port removed felt like a positive step, even though my arm was a bit painful and swollen afterwards. *Dance floor, here I come!* I thought.

But that same week, just as the horizon was looking brighter and clearer for me, disaster struck, without warning. That makes it sound really dramatic, and it wasn't, but it was still a massive blow. It was such an everyday situation: while I was walking from the living room to the kitchen I fractured the metatarsal bone in my left foot – and just like that, with a click and a quick stab of pain, my plans for dancing in the *Strictly* semi-final were shattered. I couldn't believe it! I was just so unlucky.

'What happened?' my sister asked me, when I rang her in tears, totally gutted. 'You weren't dancing, were you?'

'I was only walking!' I protested.

So it was back to the hospital, where I had a boot fitted to support and protect my foot. One of the doctors asked if I'd been experiencing any loss of feeling in my hands and feet, which is known as neuropathy and can be one of the side effects of chemo. She explained that it was probably neuropathy that had caused me to land on my foot at a strange angle and fracture it.

'It's not fair!' I said. 'I've only just rung my chemo bell and now this happens: 2023 is certainly not my year.'

She gave me a sympathetic smile. 'You'll just have to make next year twice as good to make up for it.'

But I couldn't hide my devastation. I was sick of taking it easy and now I was being forced to put my feet up again – literally. My patience was at an end, and, when I went to see a physiotherapist a few days later, I asked him, 'When can I start dancing? When can I start running?'

'You're going to have to take it gradually,' he said, which made me want to scream with frustration. More resting, more delays, more time wasted. But the physio saw it another way. 'This is probably a blessing, you know,' he went on.

I frowned, trying to hold back tears. 'How could it be a blessing?'

'Because, knowing you, you would have gone full pelt at everything. And then you could have really done some damage.'

I hung my head. He knew me too well.

'If you don't take it gradually now, you're only going to do something else – and it will probably be worse, and you'll have to wait even longer to get back to doing what you love. So, be patient and take it step by step. Otherwise, if you break something like your ankle, you might find yourself with a lifelong injury.'

OK, I thought. *I have to listen this time. It's going to kill me, but holding on a couple more months will be worth it.*

Back to the sofa I went, and within about a week my foot started to feel less tender and fragile. I went on trying to rest and recuperate, even though it drove me crazy at times, and then little by little I started doing more – I popped into the dance school, saw friends, went to a few meetings. But my sensible, patient approach to recuperation hit a wall one Monday in late November, when I began to feel poorly and started vomiting. At first, I thought it was a Crohn's flare-up, because the symptoms seemed very similar to the ones I'd experienced so many times before. But it was actually my body trying to tell me that I had another blood clot, courtesy of chemo. Thank goodness I was taking it easy because of my broken foot. Otherwise, I might have tried to carry on regardless, in typical Amy style, and then it could have been a very different story.

Within a few hours I was beginning to feel seriously unwell. I rang Ben, who was in the studio teaching. His phone was on silent, but when he checked it during a break, he noticed he'd had a missed call from me. He tried ringing back and couldn't get hold of me.

Karla was at the studio with her daughter, and Ben asked her to keep calling me while he went on teaching. When Karla couldn't get through, she got in her car to drive over. Ben had a bad feeling as well and was finding it difficult to focus, so he asked the other teachers to cover for him and made his way home a few minutes later.

When Karla arrived at our house, she found me collapsed on the floor, trying to ring Ben to say I needed help. 'Oh my God, Amy, what is it?' she asked, in a panic.

'Just feel really poorly,' I croaked, struggling to be sick.

Ben arrived to see me bringing blood up all over Karla. Luckily, I had been able to call an ambulance before I hit the floor and when the ambulance came, the paramedics tested my heart and oxygen levels. They could tell immediately that I wasn't right and rushed me into hospital. Ben came with me.

After tests at the hospital, I was sent for a CT scan on my lungs, which put me into panic mode. Had the cancer travelled to my lungs?

As I couldn't help imagining the worst when I had the tiniest twinge, you can imagine the catastrophic thoughts I was having after passing out on the floor and vomiting blood. This was serious.

'We have found something,' the doctors said when the scan came back. 'You have a blood clot on your lung and we're worried in case it's travelling to your heart.'

'What can you do?' Ben asked.

Within twenty minutes, a heart specialist and cardiology team were standing by my bed. I was already on blood thinners, which had been prescribed after I'd developed two blood clots in my arm after my second round of chemo. But they obviously weren't strong enough to prevent another blood clot, so the heart specialist felt he had no option but to put me on the strongest blood thinning medication you can get. Nobody wanted to risk a clot travelling to the heart.

Ben phoned my mum and dad, and they rushed to the hospital. I hardly registered their presence when they arrived. I felt so ill and weak – I barely woke up all day – and they said later that they thought I looked nearly as poorly as I had with the sepsis.

The hospital kept me in for a couple of days of observation and after I was discharged I had to inject myself with blood thinner every day, which made me feel sick and exhausted. And it was now, after all I'd been through, after all the obstacles and setbacks, that I reached my lowest point emotionally, I think. I was so upset, so tired of it all. I had no hair, no eyelashes; I'd broken my foot. My chemo had ended but I was almost as poorly as I'd been when I had sepsis. I was meant to be dancing on *Strictly*, and that had given me something to work towards, but now even that had been taken away from me. When was I going to get a break?

I sank so low that I couldn't imagine ever being well or happy again. I'd tried my best to be brave and keep going, to bounce back from every blow and let-down, but now, for the first time in my life, I couldn't see an end to it. Would I ever feel healthy and strong again? Would I ever be well enough to return to *Strictly*? I felt weak from constantly being knocked down and having to get up again; it was one problem after another, a succession of obstacles and disappointments, and I just felt so exhausted. I couldn't see myself getting back to what I loved again, couldn't envisage myself back on the dance floor. I felt defeated, my strength drained, my fight gone.

It felt as if everything had been stripped away, from my hair to my dancing feet, and I started to lose hope of ever being me again. When I looked in the mirror I couldn't identify myself. Where was the person I used to be, the old Amy? Was she hiding behind the sad eyes that I saw looking back at me, or had she disappeared for good? It was dark and wintry outside, reflecting the bleakness I felt inside, and I couldn't see a light anywhere. Mum and Dad were really worried about me. They'd never seen me so miserable before.

I spent my time resting, trying to recover and give myself a chance to heal physically, but a part of me just felt so bleak and hopeless. Some of my friends came to visit – Karla, Brad and Jenny all popped in, and that helped – and then Mum and Dad came to stay for a couple of nights and their love began to bring me round. It was a slow process, but over the next couple of weeks my spirits lifted slightly and I started to come out of it. I began to feel well again. I could feel my energy returning. Glimmers of hope appeared on the horizon. I was seeing my friends and trying to get a bit of my old life back.

To anyone feeling down in the depths of despair, I'd say, 'Don't hold your feelings in, let them out. If you need a good cry, have a good cry. Remember that this too shall pass and try not to lose hope. Even if you can't do what you love, surround yourself with the people you love, because it really helps. Wrap yourself around your loved ones.'

It really made a difference to me when I went down to *Strictly*, and the series producer and choreographer took me to one side in the studio. 'We've had this fabulous idea,' they said, and they asked me to appear in a dance in the grand final show. That was a massive turning point; I felt a familiar surge of determination inside me. The clot on my lung was under control and I wasn't going to get another one, because I was on the strongest blood thinners known to medical science. *That's it*, I thought. *I'm getting up and getting on with my life. Don't get bitter, get better.*

My mum and sister thought it was too soon for me to start going about like normal again, though. So who did they get to ring me and tell me I'm doing too much and need to take it easy? Carol, of course – who had straight-talked me into having chemotherapy all those months previously.

But nothing was going to stop me getting down to the *Strictly Come Dancing* final, not a broken foot and not a blood clot. I think everybody understood that in the end, especially as the amazing team at *Strictly* sorted it so that I could perform a fan dance in the opening routine, with my *Strictly* family whirling around me. The *Strictly* choreographers are just genius. They did armography and fanography with me and created something spectacular. Even though I was exhausted by the end of the evening, it gave me such a boost. Just being back there was amazing, feeling that rush of adrenalin that I'd missed so much. It made my dancing heart so happy.

A few days after the excitement had died down, Ben and I rented a little house by the sea in Wales and spent Christmas surrounded by nature. Carlos from *Strictly* joined us, and he's really fun to be around, so it turned out to be a really lovely break. It was only a few days but it was exactly what we needed after a truly terrible year: beautiful countryside, sea air and roaring fires.

Goodness, I was glad to see the back of 2023! On New Year's Eve, when everyone was posting their year's highlights, I actually felt quite bitter and jealous. At the beginning of the year, I'd had so many lovely plans. I was on the *Strictly* tour; my honeymoon with Ben was coming up; there was more filming to do on my programme, *Dare to Dance*. And then, within a day, my life changed. And it didn't just change during the treatment and recovery, it changed for ever. It changed me as a person because it stole my peace of mind. It changed my parents as well – I could tell that just by seeing the pain in their eyes. It affected all of us – my lovely husband, my dance school students, my brother and sister, my friends. I still had some amazing experiences in 2023, but when I looked back, I couldn't help feeling that I'd had almost a whole year robbed from me.

So while everyone else was sharing lovely photos and reels from their year, I was thinking, *I've had cancer, I've lost my hair and my boob, I've had sepsis, I've had blood clots and broken my foot.* And I wasn't even out of the woods yet, according to my consultant. The MRI scan of my breast had shown it to be free of cancer, which was great news. But without the results of a bone density scan, which were due a few days later, we didn't yet have a full picture of my recovery. Looking back at my journey and how things had changed along the way – at first a lumpectomy and no chemotherapy, then a mastectomy and eight chemo sessions – I didn't feel I could celebrate until all the results were back.

There was something else, too. Over Christmas I'd been having some shoulder pain and restricted shoulder movement that I knew wasn't muscular. As a dancer, I know what a muscle injury feels like, and this felt like it was in the bone. So instead of feeling like I was getting better, I tensed up again.

As the days passed and the pain didn't go away, I really started to worry. What if the cancer had spread to my bones? I realised then that I will never be able to live without worry.

Chapter 13

Make the most of every opportunity: go grab life

I couldn't stop worrying. On and on, all through the night, the what-ifs went round my head like unclaimed suitcases on a baggage carousel. My mind kept running away with all these questions: *What if I need to have more chemo? Or an operation? What if they can't do surgery until spring, and then there's six weeks recovery? How am I going to be better in time for the summer and* Strictly?

It sounds silly, but I couldn't shut it down. There was nothing I could do; my fear was constantly there, no matter what, and every day I'd be thinking and worrying about it.

The shoulder pain came on gradually over Christmas and soon I wasn't able to do any exercise – not swimming, not anything. I couldn't have danced even if I'd wanted to, and I wasn't able to anyway because I was rehabbing my foot. As I hadn't been able to exercise at all since I'd fractured my metatarsal, I knew I hadn't done anything to cause an injury to my shoulder. And that's what was worrying me, I guess.

In January, I went to see my physio. 'Something's not right,' he said, after examining my shoulder. 'And it's definitely not muscular.'

Although this only confirmed my own view, instantly I

thought, *Oh no, the cancer's spread.* That's where your mind goes to.

That same day, I had an appointment with my GP, who felt my arm and was worried it might be blood clots again. He sent me straight to A&E, where I was referred immediately to an orthopaedic doctor, who specialises in diagnosing and treating conditions that affect bones, muscles and joints.

The orthopaedic doctor was absolutely great and very understanding. He knew my history and everything I'd been through; I think he could tell I was very anxious as well, so he was completely open and honest with me. He was aware that I knew the problem wasn't muscular – I was sure it was something else, something more – and that my worry was that it was cancer.

'We need to do an MRI scan on your shoulder and check that it hasn't spread to the bones,' he said.

That put me straight into panic mode, because it's one thing to think something and another thing for a doctor to say it out loud.

I had an MRI pretty soon after that and had to wait a couple of days for the results.

I had been told that my breast was clear in December, and that was a box ticked, a relief. But even though I knew my breast was OK and I didn't need to have the other one removed, the gruelling amount of chemo that had gone into my system, and its side effects, made me feel more than ever that I was suffering from cancer. In fact, I felt more of a cancer patient than I did just after my operation; I was really emotional, really up and down, and so unsure of what the future might hold.

By now, people were asking when I would find out if the chemo had worked. 'Weren't you having your final scan in December?'

'Just waiting for the last of the results,' I said, as lightly as I could.

I didn't want to worry everyone, after they'd already been so worried, so the only people who were aware of my concerns were my parents, Ben and my sister. When you don't know something, you don't want to panic people unnecessarily. I didn't have anything to update them with, so I thought, *Let's just keep this quiet and deal with it when we know.*

I think this is the reality now, for me – such is the anxiety behind any pain or niggle that your mind instantly jumps to thinking, *Is it cancer?* Jenny had told me about this: any little lump – any anything – triggers the anxiety that is there. Already I was experiencing it for myself. I think it's going to be something that I have to learn to live with.

This is why I keep wanting to put out the message: *You know your own body, so if you think there is something wrong, don't rest on it. Go and get it checked out.* I can't stress that enough.

You don't get mammograms until you're in your fifties, so if you're not checking, who is? If I hadn't started checking my chest after the CoppaFeel charity trek in 2022, I dread to think what my outcome would have been, because my breast cancer was grade three out of three, the most aggressive type. So I'm on a mission now to get that message across to people. I did my first CoppaFeel charity trek almost one year to the day before I had my mastectomy. The next trek I'm doing will be exactly a year after the mastectomy, and again I'll be trekking to raise awareness, raise money for CoppaFeel and remind people to check their chests. I feel I've come full circle.

✦

I was terrified when the doctor phoned me with results of the MRI scan. The gap between potential good news and potential bad news was so enormous that I could barely bring myself to answer his call. It felt like life or death. I was confident about my breast, but with my bone, I had no idea, so when he said, 'We've found something', my heart plunged.

Then he said, 'But it's not cancer,' and I burst into tears.

Oh my God! I thought, as the weight of months of worry lifted off me and floated away.

'It's an impingement, but we can deal with it; don't panic,' he went on, but after hearing there was no cancer, I didn't care what he said – I was just delighted.

An impingement is when a tendon in your shoulder rubs or catches on the bone, causing pain as you lift your arm. You can treat it with steroid injections or physiotherapy, and I'm going down the physio route to begin with. Injections are the next level and the worst-case scenario is surgery.

What caused it? Chemo could have caused it, or the overuse of my shoulder from dancing. It's very rare to have an impingement on the shoulder at my age – it normally comes a lot later in life – but still it's a far better outcome than the one I feared. If cancer was in my bone, that would be secondary cancer, which is stage four and terminal. Impingement is nothing on that.

I instantly rang Ben. He had been quietly confident that we'd have good news but didn't want to jinx anything by actually saying it. 'You knew something was wrong,' he said. 'But you were thinking the worst!'

I couldn't wait to hug him. He'd been so positive all along, so supportive.

A couple of days later, I went to see the doctor to get the final results of all my scans and tests. When I came out, I had a really good cry with my sister. 'You've done it, you're through it. You can put all this behind you,' she kept saying.

It was the biggest sense of relief. *We've made it*, we thought.

At the moment, I've got no evidence of disease, which is amazing. I won't get an all-clear for five years, because of the type of cancer I've had – a hormone-fed cancer – and I'll need an injection once a month and regular check-ups. But it's the best outcome I could have hoped for.

Had they found more cancer or said I needed more chemo, or more surgery, then I might not have been able to do *Strictly* this year. And if I'd needed to have my other breast off, it would have taken away the chance of ever being able to breastfeed a baby. So it really was the best news.

I'm like a different person now. I can't stop smiling, laughing and giggling. It's amazing to go to sleep without that voice in the back of my mind asking, *But what if this . . . and what if that . . . ?* I can just put my head on the pillow and I'm off.

My foot slowly improved and by March I was hopping on it. I wasn't rushing my recovery, though. At long last, I had learned my lesson and was being patient so that I didn't overdo it and end up taking a step backwards. Maybe I didn't mention to my physiotherapist that I was doing the odd bit of teaching here and there, but slowly and surely, things were going the right way and I was planning to be dancing again by Easter.

Yes, I've learned to be patient for the first time in my life! Maybe I've said that before, but in the past, I always used to have to learn the hard way. It was the sepsis that started to turn it around, I think. That's when I learned how serious it could be if I did too much too quickly – when I realised it could be a matter of life and death, in fact, and it was crucial to approach my recovery properly. And after I broke my foot, I realised again, *Yeah, I really do have to listen to my body.* Otherwise, I'm just going to face more and more setbacks.

I know 100 per cent that my fractured metatarsal was the universe telling me to slow down! Had I gone back straight to dancing – and I wanted to, even though I clearly wasn't in the place to be able to – I could have broken my back or injured myself in another major way. Everybody's telling me the same thing: it was definitely a warning.

Along with patience, I've learned that, at times like this, you find out who your true family and friends are. It's been a bit of a hard learning curve, because, as I mentioned, some people I might have expected to support me haven't been there, and that's been quite tough. But I can also see that I truly do have the best family and friends around me; I have learned to spend as much time as I can with my loved ones, and to tell them I love them every day. I've been given a second chance at life now, and I'm very aware that others haven't – I'm thinking of my friend and pink sister Nicky, who sadly passed away in 2023. Unfortunately, breast cancer took Nicky and I'm determined now to go by the motto she lived by. I even had it printed on a T-shirt that I wore on the day I finished chemo: GO GRAB LIFE.

I thought of Nicky when I was given the good news about my scans and test results. I was like, *OK, I'm done. Here we go. Go grab life.* Yet again, I have known what it's like to have my dancing taken away from me, so I just want to make the most of dancing and any opportunity that comes my way.

Something important I've realised on this journey is that beauty comes from within, not from the exterior. I had everything stripped away from me: my hair, my eyelashes and eyebrows; I gained two stone in weight from taking steroids. In time, I learned to think, *You know what? This is what my body needs to go through right now in order to survive.*

I'm so relieved for my parents that it's all over, too. Getting the final results means my dad is able to go to bed now and sleep at night. I know both Mum and Dad really struggled during my course of treatment, especially after the sepsis and blood clot episodes; and they struggled when I was first diagnosed, as well. Dad had to take time off work because of stress, and it's been tough for my mum, because she's had breast cancer herself, so she knows some of what I've had to go through. On top of this, the sepsis brought back the shock and sadness of losing her sister, my aunt. So my parents have had to go through a lot of trauma and, to be honest, I think it'll take a bit of time for them to fully recover.

As for Ben, my wonderful husband, everyone is saying how happy he is. We're both in a good place now; we've been able to exhale and relax at last. We're planning to do everything that we planned to do in 2023 but couldn't, so we're in full swing with the house renovations, we're really busy with the dance studio and planning a holiday. We're able to see the future now. Life is resuming for us and we're taking it a day at a time. In a couple of years we'll hopefully look at our fertility options again, but for now we're focusing on getting me better.

✦

I've been so, so lucky; Ben has just been the most amazing help and support throughout this time. Of course, I don't ever need to be reminded of what an amazing human being he is, but then the team at ITV's *Lorraine* sent us away on holiday to the Caribbean island of Grenada, and I realised it all over again. It was like another honeymoon for us, a lovely trip that they wanted us to experience to make up for our actual honeymoon, which was overshadowed by my silent fixation on what the lump in my breast could be.

So we were whisked away to this beautiful island, with its gorgeous beaches and clear blue sea, and while we were there we realised that we needed a break more than we could possibly have imagined. It was lovely to have quality time together and not be worrying about getting to hospital appointments – bearing in mind that I'd had seven of them in the week before we left. Getting away from all of that was just wonderful, and being able to switch off and relax, something neither of us had been able to do for a long time. Ben had been working so hard all year, looking after me in every way while spinning plates to keep the dance studio going, and although I'd had loads of time doing nothing, I'd not really had a chance to relax – and for me the best way to unwind is to listen to the sea.

It was just what we needed – it was heavenly to have the music on as we sat and played Uno, chilling by the pool, or to go to the spa and have a head massage or some other lush treatment. Ben loves being pampered even more than I do! We did some really cool things: we went on a boat trip and jumped off the deck into the warm, clear water; we made chocolate bars at a chocolate factory; we tasted different types of rum and had some fantastic meals at the beach. We did everything that we've missed out on, I guess. Most of all, it was so amazing to have that time together.

Having those few days of sunshine helped push my recovery forward. At the time of writing, it's going well and I'm feeling so much better day by day. The fatigue is getting better, my hair is growing back and my foot is healing. I am definitely coming out of the side effects of chemo. I'm still having to inject myself every day because of my blood clots, but I'm definitely feeling stronger and brighter.

I was already a survivor when I discovered I had breast cancer. Having Crohn's disease had toughened me up. But nothing could have prepared me for the turbulent weeks and months of my cancer journey, especially the emotional side of it, and I think it's going to take some time for me to get over it, if I'm honest. It still feels very surreal when I think about what I've been through; I'm still processing and digesting it all now, and I have to accept that it's going to be very much part of my life for the next several years. It's about learning to live with it, in the weirdest of ways, but it's going to take a while because I've been through so much and so much has happened to my body. I've got a new body – I've got new scars – and I don't think I fully accept that yet. But I know that one day all of it will be a distant memory.

My Crohn's has been fine, touch wood; I'll be very careful about my diet and hopefully I won't have any nasty flare-ups, as I'm not sure I could cope with that right now. In a way, and I never thought this would happen, my Crohn's disease has taken a back seat. Or if not a back seat, a seat to the side. Since I was eleven, it has been the priority when it comes to my health, so it's been really strange to find that hasn't been the case recently, because saving my life overtook it as my priority. Maybe now I can learn to continue not to worry as much about Crohn's as I used to. It was always such a source of anxiety in the past, and maybe it doesn't need to be.

People often say that you should have a positive attitude through cancer. But I don't think there's a textbook on how to deal with a cancer diagnosis. You just have to do what's right for you. I've been very open and honest about it and spoken about it, but that approach doesn't work for everyone. Some people shave their hair off when they start chemo, whereas I wanted to cling on to my hair for as long as I possibly could and then took the decision halfway through that I couldn't cope and wanted to take control. There's no right or wrong way. You've got to deal with it in a way that works for you.

Another thing people say is that you've got to be strong. Well, there were moments where I was strong, but there were also moments where I really wasn't, and that is OK, too. I guess it's about learning to accept all the emotions that you do go through, and knowing it's all right to feel like this.

I cried a lot. The best piece of advice I could have had at

the beginning of the journey, I think, was from my specialist cancer nurse: 'Cry and let it out. Don't let it build up.'

What else has got me through? Really? It's the strength and determination that my parents taught me from a young age. It's the love and support Ben has given me, and his positivity. It's our dear friends. Seeing my pink sister Jenny come out the other side of breast cancer, and go on to live her life to the full, was a daily reminder that I could get better too. Also having *Strictly* there and still feeling a part of it – I'm not sure how I would have coped if I hadn't got to go down to *Strictly* when I was well.

After every chemo, when I was feeling desperately poorly, I'd say to myself, I'm going to get better so that I can get down to *Strictly* next weekend.

It gave me something to work towards, and when I was there, it was the reminder I needed that this was worth fighting for.

I'm going to get through the bad times so that I can get back to doing what I love most, I vowed. One day I'd love to win *Strictly*, but winning for me would be being back with the gang, doing what I love in front of the audience with the people I love.

Before I had the news that my body was free of cancer, I couldn't help thinking, *Is there going to be any point?* Now I just feel free. I feel like I can plan, I can look ahead. I've got the spring back in my step; I've got my motivation back.

Now that I can see that I've got a whole life to live and I've been given a second chance, I'm just going to grab every opportunity I possibly can.

I just want to get back on that dance floor. I've missed it so much. I've been able to do a bit of teaching. I've been watching competitions. I've been planning and choreographing ideas in my head, and I'll be able to dance again soon. But I haven't been able to do any performing – I can't wait to be able to perform up close and personal to an audience again. It's going to make my heart happy. And that's when I'm going feel like I'm really back to being me again.

I'm so grateful for another chance at life.

Epilogue

Friday, 14 June 2024. I'm lying on the sofa, my legs heavily strapped. My blistered toes peep above the laptop, each one a reminder of an emotional and physically demanding 100km trek in the Brecon Beacons for CoppaFeel!. As I type this, I reflect on how much my life has changed in the two years since my first CoppaFeel! trek. It was that trek which led me to start checking myself and, ultimately, saved my life. It's a year since my mastectomy. And now I had trekked again, to give back to the charity that did so much for me, helping to raise funds and awareness so that hopefully, one day, no one will be left unchecked.

This trek was so much harder than my first. It is clear to me that my body is not yet what it was. Whereas once I could've walked all day and danced all night, my muscles and joints ache, my skin sore. I've come so far but still have some way to go before I'm in the shape I would want to be for a gruelling *Strictly* season.

I'm tired and emotional, but so happy – the joy of crossing the finish line less than 24 hours ago still within me. With my Pink Sister Jenny with me too, it was quite the week. Reflecting and supporting each other, as we did throughout our cancer journey. I was a team captain for thirty-one incredible ladies whose stories touched my heart. Together we laughed, we cried and pushed each other during the times when we didn't feel like we could continue. Of course, our daily 7am warm-ups included dancing and the hokey cokey. A new group of beautiful friends, for ever bonded by this experience.

As we came closer to the finish line my emotions came through stronger than ever. I guess being away from everyday life, having time to think, reflecting on the last two years all came pouring out. Giovanna Fletcher looked at me and knew I needed to get my head down at certain times, knew when to tap my shoulder for support, to tell me how proud she was, how she loved me and hold my hand.

We walked up, leading the group to the finish line with Jenny just slightly behind. I had the biggest smile, through tears of emotion, gratitude and pride. Giovanna and I grabbed each other, cried together and it felt like I was stepping out from the past year of that horrendous journey to better times ahead. I felt I owed it all to Gi. I also felt stronger in myself – that the new me, my new body, got through this.

It's been a special week. In that way the universe works sometimes, everything seems to have aligned, the disparate strands of my journey coming together. Away from the trek, it was announced I would be returning to *Strictly* and in just a couple of days I will be returning to the dancefloor for the first time in twelve months, dancing with my husband Ben, making it even more special. I look at my toes again; no amount of blisters is going to stop me getting my dancing shoes back on for that.

I'm also nervously excited for tonight, because I can finally reveal the secret I've been carrying around with me for the past month (which has not been easy!). I can't quite believe it. I don't think I ever will. At 10.30pm on this day the King's Birthday Honours are released and my name is on it. I have been made a Member of the Order of the British Empire. Amy Dowden MBE. I've been recognised for my work raising awareness of Crohn's and inflammatory bowel disease. I'm still in shock, but it has given me even more inspiration to continue advocating for more awareness and research into this terrible chronic illness.

How did that little girl with enormous dreams end up on the biggest entertainment show, and have the privilege and honour of an MBE? What a difference a year can make. Forever grateful.

You become who you surround yourself with. I know I have the best family and group of friends around me. I'm proud to be an ambassador for amazing charities. As I gaze at the rain outside the window, I'm starting to daydream less about my cancer returning and more about returning to *Strictly*, and of course visiting the palace to accept my MBE. Once I would've been frustrated by the rain, now I just want to dance in it.

Acknowledgements

Thank you . . .

Jillian Young, my editor at Little, Brown: for giving me the opportunity to share my story and hopefully help others. Rebecca Cripps: for bringing my story to life and making a dream come true. Andrew Wilson and Abigail Owens, my agents, for your guidance and support, and Morwenna Loughman, my literary agent.

All the doctors and nurses who have cared for me. Crohns and Colitis UK, the charity dedicated to helping people with inflammatory bowel disease, and CoppaFeel, the breast cancer charity that saved my life.

Strictly Come Dancing for inspiring my dance journey and my *Strictly* family for always believing in me.

Ben's parents, Simon and Elaine, who were so supportive of our dream to become British champions. My mum and dad, my brother and sister, and my friends, who have all been amazing, with a special thanks to Jenny and Karla, for everything you've done: Ben and I couldn't have got through this past year without you.

And, finally, to my one and only Ben, I can't wait to share the future with you.

Resources

Here are some contacts you might find useful:

CROHN'S AND COLITIS

Crohn's and Colitis UK

https://crohnsandcolitis.org.uk/
Helpline: 0300 222 5700
Email: helpline@crohnsandcolitis.org.uk
Live chat: https://crohnsandcolitis.org.uk/info-support/
support-for-you

Guts UK

Research and campaigning to raise awareness about
digestive disorders.
https://gutscharity.org.uk/

BREAST CANCER AWARENESS

CoppaFeel is a breast cancer awareness charity with a mission to educate and remind every young person in the UK to check their breasts regularly. There's lots of info and advice about how to contact your GP and what happens next if you notice an unusual change in your chest. https://coppafeel.org/

The **NHS** website has a resources page for people affected by breast cancer. https://www.nhs.uk/conditions/breast-cancer-in-women/ help-and-support-for-breast-cancer-in-women/

Breast Cancer Now

https://breastcancernow.org
Helpline: 0808 800 6000

Macmillan Cancer Support

https://www.macmillan.org.uk/
(where you can access specialist online support and a breast cancer forum)
Free support line: 0808 808 00 00

HEALTH/HOSPITAL ADVOCACY

An advocate is an independent professional who is on your side. They can explain your options to you, help you decide what you want and support you to have your say and know your rights. Advocates don't work for the council, the NHS, or care providers.

Some hospitals and GP practices will be able to direct you to an advocacy service, so enquire locally. You can also contact social care services at your local council and ask about advocacy services.

The Fremantle Trust website has information about the different types of advocacy and how to access them.
https://www.fremantletrust.org/help-and-advice/what-is-an-advocate-in-health-and-social-care-and-what-is-their-role?
Info line: 01296 393000
Email: enquiries@fremantletrust.org

The Advocacy People can offer advice on how to find someone to help you make your voice heard in a healthcare setting, and to raise concerns or make a complaint about an NHS service.
https://www.theadvocacypeople.org.uk/
Info line: 0330 440 9000

VoiceAbility offers free, independent support in having your say and knowing your rights.
Call 0300 303 1660 (Mon–Fri, 9–5) or email helpline@voiceability.org
They can help you find out if you are eligible for an advocate service and what is available in your area.